T0276028

THE FOUNDATION FOR FACIAL RECOVERY

FIX MY FACE

Expert Advice for Maximizing Recovery from Bell's Palsy, Ramsay Hunt Syndrome, and Other Causes of Facial Nerve Paralysis

Copyright © 2020 The Foundation for Facial Recovery

All rights reserved. No part of this book may be used or reproduced by any means, graphic, electronic, or mechanical, including photocopying, recording, taping or by any information storage retrieval system without the written permission of the author except in the case of brief quotations embodied in critical articles and reviews.

This book contains information about Bell's palsy, Ramsay Hunt syndrome, and other facial paralysis caused by viral and acquired means. It presents background information, standard and unique physical therapy treatment interventions, plastic surgery options, and other interventions being used by healthcare professionals to treat facial palsy. However, this book is not intended to replace the advice of a licensed physician or healthcare professional.

No actual person is discussed in this book.

Damages of any kind—whether commercial or personal—resulting from the use of information in this book will not be the responsibility of the author. "The author" shall include editorial contributors and The Foundation for Facial Recovery.

Considerable effort has been taken to corroborate the accuracy of statements in this text; however, neither the publisher nor any of the parties involved in the creation of this book guarantee the validity of the information. Additionally, its use by readers should be restricted to educational purposes only as a review of available treatment options. Suggestions presented here regarding current treatment modalities should not be employed unless discussed with a qualified healthcare professional.

Mention in this book does not imply the authors' endorsement or promotion of individual medical procedures, diagnostic tests, products, or treatments.

Medical research, studies, protocols, and guidelines surrounding facial palsy continue to evolve, making the information in this book subject to change. Before embarking on any regimen outlined here—whether pertaining to medication, therapies, or lifestyle—please consult with a licensed healthcare professional for clearance.

Diagnosis of, and treatment for, any condition is within the purview of licensed or certified healthcare professionals and should not be undertaken by individuals simply based on what they have read here. We encourage you to consult with practicing medical professionals concerning your specific condition.

By reading this disclaimer, you are assumed to acquiesce to these stipulations before reading the book.

iUniverse books may be ordered through booksellers or by contacting:

iUniverse
1663 Liberty Drive
Bloomington, IN 47403
www.iuniverse.com
1-800-Authors (1-800-288-4677)

Because of the dynamic nature of the Internet, any web addresses or links contained in this book may have changed since publication and may no longer be valid. The views expressed in this work are solely those of the author and do not necessarily reflect the views of the publisher, and the publisher hereby disclaims any responsibility for them.

ISBN: 978-1-5320-9159-9 (sc)
ISBN: 978-1-5320-9160-5 (e)

Library of Congress Control Number: 2020906146

Print information available on the last page.

iUniverse rev. date: 06/23/2020

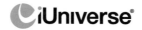

DEDICATION

This book is dedicated to the many patients with facial palsy who have given us the privilege of accompanying them on their journey to healing. They truly inspire and motivate us every day.

INTRODUCTION

With this book in your hands, chances are you've just been diagnosed with Bell's palsy or have been dealing with its disheartening effects for some time now. Or perhaps you've been struggling with facial paralysis for months or even years due to a tumor, surgery, Lyme disease, or some other cause.

Regardless, we know how devastating it can be to see a stranger looking back in the mirror, to have a photo taken, to simply try to blink, speak clearly, or eat and drink as effortlessly as you once did.

Most of all, we know you are hoping that there's something, *anything* out there to help restore the face you once knew.

As physical therapists who work with facial palsy patients every day and collaborate with a multidisciplinary team of facial nerve specialists, we're here to tell you *there is*.

Pharmaceuticals taken at onset, specialized physical therapy, plastic surgery, and other modalities can form a powerful partnership to significantly improve facial appearance and function in nearly everyone with facial paralysis or weakness.

This is possible even if you've been told by one or more healthcare professionals that all you can do is wait to see if you'll get better.

This is possible even if you've been told you're just not going to improve … that this is "your new normal."

This is possible even if you've been living with facial palsy for many years.

These are bold statements and likely welcome news for many of the frontline healthcare providers who see people with sudden facial paralysis in those first panicked hours or days.

Even though Bell's palsy strikes some 40,000 people each year in the United States alone, the malady is not fully understood or even very familiar to many. Medical experts know what happens to nerves and muscles in the face when sudden facial paralysis occurs, and most now agree reactivation of a dormant ("sleeping") virus in the body is most likely to blame. But what causes that virus to "wake up" and wreak havoc to begin with, and why? Lacking empirical evidence, we can only cite correlations: pregnancy and diabetes are two factors that seem to put people at risk, for example, but so do more intangible considerations such as stress and a weakened immune system.

The diagnosis of facial palsy suffers from a lack of urgency in the medical community. Approximately 70 percent of people will experience full or nearly complete healing spontaneously, typically within a few weeks to three months, or up to a year at the outside. (That's great news for those of you in the early days of paralysis!) As a result, treatment options for the comparatively small cohort of patients who have lingering deficits and complications haven't been widely and scientifically pursued.

But finding ways to conquer facial palsy is urgent to us!

As the principal clinicians behind The Center for Facial Recovery and its nonprofit arm, The Foundation for Facial Recovery, in Rockville, Maryland, we are among the few physical therapists anywhere passionately developing effective interventions for facial palsy while also educating healthcare providers and the public about the condition. Through our years of experience, we've helped thousands of patients with facial challenges.

Even better, by partnering with a team of top experts in facial plastic surgery, oculoplastic surgery, dentistry, biofeedback, and other specialties—and by building upon current standards of care and clinical-based evidence—we have developed an approach to tackling facial palsy that is proving to be as effective as it is unique.

What we've learned lies at the heart of this book.

What do we want *you* to learn from these pages? First, that you're not alone. That we understand both your physical pain and the very real, complex loss and emotional pain that no one you know can truly understand if they haven't gone through it themselves.

Our goal with *Fix My Face* is to give you what has no doubt been elusive until now: one authoritative source of comprehensive information you can trust.

Along with a thorough understanding of your condition, we'll suggest an action plan for healing that you can discuss with your physician. You will come away with

- advice on when and how to seek out professionals who specialize in facial nerve disorders.
- a look at exciting, innovative treatments that are making a real difference for patients.
- plastic surgery procedures that can improve appearance and facial function.
- cautions about so-called "treatments" that can worsen your condition.
- mental strategies to help you face the world with more confidence.

From one of the first patients we ever saw with Bell's palsy—a mother who was stricken while pregnant and couldn't bear to be photographed with her baby—to the most recent ones to walk through our door, we see and feel the emotions that pour out during sessions. We honor the very real grief with slow recoveries and celebrate the victories when someone's eye resumes closing by itself or their smile begins to open up.

But the greatest inspiration behind what we do, and the best assurance we can give to you, comes from the surprising strength we see in nearly everyone with facial palsy. In our experience, these individuals are by far the hardest-working, most determined clients once they learn that this condition responds to diligent effort, be it through performing facial exercises at home or persevering in the search for a qualified specialist who can provide an adjunct procedure or treatment. We're confident that you, too, will have the fortitude and resourcefulness to meet this challenge, whether you're facing it short-term or for an extended period.

So read on, have faith—and smile. You're going to get better.

--Jodi M. Barth, PT, CCI
Cofounder, The Center for Facial Recovery, Rockville, Maryland
President and board member, The Foundation for Facial Recovery
--Gincy L. Stezar, PTA, CCI
Cofounder, The Center for Facial Recovery
Secretary and board member, The Foundation for Facial Recovery

TABLE OF CONTENTS

CONTRIBUTORS

This book is made possible by support from The J. Willard and Alice S. Marriott Foundation

Jodi Maron Barth, PT, CCI

Jodi Barth is cofounder of The Center for Facial Recovery in Rockville, Maryland, and president of The Foundation for Facial Recovery. She is one of only a handful of recognized facial palsy therapists in the United States. She is a licensed physical therapist with 40 years of experience in the field of rehabilitation with a specialization in outpatient rehabilitation.

Jodi's wide range of clinical experience has provided her with the tools to perform in-depth, comprehensive physical therapy evaluations and treatments using dry needling, graded motor imagery, biofeedback, extensive manual therapy, TMJ Rocabado techniques, and more. She is a sought-after speaker nationally and internationally in the areas of TMD (jaw symptoms), facial palsy, postural dysfunction, and performance enhancement for the vocal artist.

Jodi is a published author and certified clinical instructor through the American Physical Therapy Association (APTA) and has served on the APTA House of Delegates for the past three years. She is also a faculty research assistant at the University of Maryland. Jodi is a graduate of the Ithaca College PT program and attended the Master of Science program at Adelphi University in the area of exercise physiology.

Lauren Mills Bolding, DDS

Dr. Lauren Mills Bolding is a clinical associate in the Johns Hopkins Department of Otolaryngology–Head and Neck Surgery. She received her Doctor of Dental Surgery degree from New York University in 2009 and completed the prosthodontics residency program at the University of Maryland Baltimore in 2012. Then, Dr. Bolding completed a one-year fellowship at the Memorial Sloan-Kettering Cancer Center focusing on maxillofacial prosthetics and dental oncology.

A board-certified prosthodontist, Dr. Bolding treats patients with oral and maxillofacial cancer. Her other areas of expertise include maxillofacial prosthetics, cosmetic dentistry, restorative dentistry, and TMD. She is on the board of directors of The Foundation for Facial Recovery.

Carl Chua, PT, CCI

Carl Chua is a licensed physical therapist with more than 15 years of experience working in the outpatient setting, primarily in orthopedic and sports rehabilitation. Carl has a comprehensive treatment approach when it comes to his patients. He uses a multitude of interventions, from Rocabado techniques for TMD, facial neuromuscular retraining, strain/counter-strain, dry needling, muscle energy techniques, myofascial release, movement screens, functional strengthening, and taping to heal his patients and return them to their full potential. Carl has also presented at various conferences both nationally and internationally on facial palsy, TMD, and spine disorders.

He is a graduate of the physical therapy program of the University of Santo Tomas. He is also a certified clinical instructor through the American Physical Therapy Association.

Christine M. Clark, MD

Dr. Christine M. Clark is currently a third-year resident physician in the Department of Otolaryngology–Head and Neck Surgery at MedStar Georgetown University Hospital. She completed her undergraduate work at the University of Pittsburgh in 2011 and spent a year teaching adult literacy classes through AmeriCorps. She then received her medical degree from Penn State University College of Medicine, where she founded a student-run free clinic for medically underserved residents of central Pennsylvania. Dr. Clark's clinical interests include the management of facial paralysis, quality improvement initiatives, medical student education, and outcomes-based research.

Betsy D. Hirschel, LCSW-C

Betsy Hirschel is a licensed certified social worker and psychotherapist in Bethesda, Maryland. She has been in private practice for more than 25 years working with individuals, couples, and groups around such topics as grief, loss, relationships, and trauma. She has postgraduate training in each of these fields of study. She also has conducted trainings in grief and loss for several law firms and corporations.

Betsy's career began as an elementary school teacher in Montgomery County, Maryland. Subsequently, she worked in parenting education and has written several study guides for running infant and toddler parenting programs. Betsy also has worked in the field of adoption, incorporating her training in infertility and neonatal and postnatal death.

After serving as president of a local chapter of Resolve (a national infertility support organization), she became the mental health director for the national Resolve organization. Several of her articles have been published in their journal. Betsy has written and presented several studies to a wide variety of organizations, including Holy Cross Hospital, the Jewish Community Center of Greater Washington, the American Fertility and Reproductive Society, and The Catholic University in Washington, DC.

Betsy is on the board of directors of The Foundation for Facial Recovery.

Emily Perlman, MS, LCPC, BCB, SMC-C

Emily Perlman is a fellow with the Biofeedback Certification International Alliance as well as a certified stress management consultant with the American Institute of Health Care Professionals. She began her 35-year career working in the field of mental health at Walter Reed Army Medical Center and at George Washington University. Sixteen years ago, Emily incorporated biofeedback into her practice and has since expanded her areas of expertise to include muscle reeducation for pain management and heart rate variability (HRV) biofeedback for stress-related disorders. Individually, or in combination, these types of biofeedback can be highly effective for clients with stress-related conditions, migraines, and other chronic pain disorders.

Emily completed two Master of Science degrees: one from the University of North Carolina at Chapel Hill and the other in mental health counseling from Walden University. She is a licensed clinical professional counselor in the State of Maryland. Additionally, she is a published author and was a principal neurofeedback therapist in Chicago's Rush Presbyterian-St. Luke's Medical Center's fibromyalgia study.

Richard Redett, MD

Dr. Richard Redett is a professor of plastic and reconstructive surgery and pediatrics at the Johns Hopkins University School of Medicine. His areas of clinical expertise include pediatric plastic surgery, cleft lip and palate surgery, obstetric brachial plexus palsy reconstruction, facial paralysis, pediatric burn surgery and reconstruction, and genital reconstruction.

Dr. Redett serves as the director of the Cleft and Craniofacial Center, the director of the Facial Paralysis and Pain Center, and the director of pediatric plastic surgery at the Johns Hopkins School of Medicine. He is also a codirector of the Brachial Plexus Clinic at the Kennedy Krieger Institute. Dr. Redett directs the genital transplant program at Johns Hopkins.

He graduated from Dartmouth Medical School after earning his undergraduate degrees in biology and psychology at Emory University. He did his general surgery and plastic surgery training at the Johns Hopkins Hospital.

Dr. Redett lectures nationally on facial paralysis, genital reconstruction, and many pediatric plastic surgery topics. He is a member of the American Cleft Palate–Craniofacial Association, the American Association of Plastic Surgeons, and the American Society of Plastic Surgeons.

Dr. Redett has a strong commitment to international health and has done many teaching medical missions to Central and South America and Africa. He serves on the board of ReSurge International, a not-for-profit organization that provides reconstructive surgical care for children and adults.

Michael J. Reilly, MD

Dr. Michael J. Reilly is an associate professor of facial plastic and reconstructive surgery in the Department of Otolaryngology–Head and Neck Surgery at Medstar Georgetown University Hospital. Dr. Reilly received his medical degree from the University of North Carolina, followed by a residency in otolaryngology–head and neck surgery at MedStar Georgetown University Hospital. After completing a fellowship in facial plastic and reconstructive surgery at the University of California Los Angeles Medical Center, in 2009 Dr. Reilly joined the same department where he completed his residency. He is double board-certified in otolaryngology–head and neck surgery, and facial plastic and reconstructive surgery.

His clinical interests include facial reanimation after facial nerve damage, repair of facial deformities, facial rejuvenation, microvascular reconstruction for head and neck cancer defects, melanoma of the head and neck, and functional and cosmetic rhinoplasty and sinus surgery. Dr. Reilly's research interests include the use of information technology to improve patient satisfaction and resident education; gender differences in facial aesthetics; and the role of physical therapy in facial rehabilitation. He has published novel research investigating how patients are perceived differently after facial surgery. His work has garnered national attention, including appearances on NBC, Fox, and *The Today Show*. In addition to his clinical practice, Dr. Reilly has an active role educating medical students and resident physicians.

Dr. Reilly is a founding board member of The Foundation for Facial Recovery.

Clayton Shiu, LAc, PhD

Dr. Clayton Shiu has been in practice for more than 20 years in the New York City medical community. He specializes in the treatment of stroke and cerebral and neurological disorders.

In 2013, Dr. Shiu was awarded a special scholarship by the Chinese government to study at Tianjin University of Traditional Chinese Medicine, where he received his Doctorate of Philosophy in acupuncture and moxibustion. In Tianjin, Dr. Shiu interned directly under his mentor, Dr. Shi Xue Min, the pioneer of stroke therapy and creator of the Xing Nao Kai Qiao (XNKQ) "Awaken the Spirit and Open the Orifice" System. Dr. Shiu assisted with treating patients at the First Teaching Hospital of Tianjin, the largest acupuncture and moxibustion stroke medical center in China. After studying in China, he created a new system called Nanopuncture®, which utilizes key components of XNKQ combined with PNF stretching and myofascial sports techniques for the treatment of stroke and orthopedic rehabilitation. Dr. Shiu teaches the Nanopuncture® educational system across the nation to assist in treating stroke, Parkinson's, and TBI disorders.

Dr. Shiu is currently an adjunct faculty professor at the American College of Traditional Chinese Medicine and the Academy of Chinese Culture and Health Sciences. He is also a founding member of the Neuroscience Acupuncture Summit.

Gincy Lockhart Stezar, PTA, CCI

Gincy Stezar is cofounder of The Center for Facial Recovery in Rockville, Maryland, and vice president/secretary of The Foundation for Facial Recovery. She is a licensed physical therapist assistant with more than 18 years of experience in the field of rehabilitation. For the past 16 years, she has collaborated with Jodi M. Barth, PT, CCI, specializing in facial neuromuscular retraining, postural restoration, and TMD. Prior to that, Gincy worked for eight years at NASA Goddard Space Flight Center as the clinic fitness director.

Gincy has presented both nationally and internationally on facial palsy, postural restoration, graded motor imagery, and TMD rehabilitation. She is a certified clinical instructor through the American Physical Therapy Association (APTA) and is presently serving as an alternate to the APTA House of Delegates. She is also a faculty research assistant at the University of Maryland. Gincy earned her Bachelor of Science degree in physical education from the University of Maryland, as well as an associate degree in applied science as a physical therapist assistant at Montgomery College.

Kalpesh Vakharia, MD, MS

Dr. Kalpesh Vakharia is associate professor of otorhinolaryngology–head and neck surgery, chief of facial plastic and reconstructive surgery, and director of the Facial Nerve Center at the University of Maryland Department of Otorhinolaryngology–Head and Neck Surgery.

Dr. Vakharia is double board-certified in facial plastic and reconstructive surgery and otolaryngology. He earned undergraduate degrees in biochemistry and computer science and engineering from the University of Pennsylvania in 2001. He also earned a Master of Science in chemistry at the University of Pennsylvania in 2001. He went on to complete his medical degree at the University of California, San Francisco, in 2006. He completed a general surgical internship at Brigham and Women's Hospital in 2007. He then joined the Harvard Medical School Otolaryngology Residency Program and completed residency training in otolaryngology in 2011. Thereafter, he completed a fellowship in facial plastic and reconstructive surgery at the Cleveland Clinic in 2012. After completing the fellowship, he joined the University of Maryland Department of Otorhinolaryngology–Head and Neck Surgery.

An expert in both surgical and nonsurgical techniques of facial rejuvenation and reconstruction, his areas of interest include cosmetic and functional surgery of the nose, eyelids and brows, skin cancer and trauma reconstruction, head and neck reconstruction, microvascular reconstruction, and the treatment of facial paralysis.

Nathan Yokel, MD

Dr. Nathan Yokel completed his undergraduate degree at the University of Maryland followed by medical school at the University of Pennsylvania. He augmented his medical training with master's degrees in public health and business administration at Johns Hopkins University. Dr. Yokel completed his internship at Union Memorial Hospital in Baltimore. He completed his residency training in physical medicine and rehabilitation with a focus on diagnostic and interventional ultrasound and sports medicine at the Georgetown University Hospital/National Rehabilitation Hospital training program, serving as chief resident in his final year and developing a research protocol for assessing the accuracy of ultrasound-guided injections. Following residency, he trained in interventional spinal procedures, regenerative procedures, and pain and occupational medicine.

Dr. Yokel believes in an integrated approach that begins with a careful review of the history of the injury or pain. He then incorporates traditional physical examination and real-time ultrasound to determine the exact cause of each individual patient's pain or impaired function. His focus on sports medicine and regenerative treatments, as well as traditional procedures and rehabilitation, combine to help patients get back to the activities they enjoy most.

Chad Zatezalo, MD

Dr. Chad Zatezalo is a fellow of the American Society of Ophthalmic Plastic and Reconstructive Surgeons and the American Academy of Ophthalmology. He specializes exclusively in plastic, reconstructive, and cosmetic surgery of the eyelids, surrounding tissue, and upper face in addition to ophthalmology. His training in both oculofacial plastics and ophthalmology allows him to understand the importance of the functional aspect of the eyelid and upper face while performing cosmetic surgery.

Dr. Zatezalo completed a two-year accredited ASOPRS fellowship at the renowned Bascom Palmer Eye Institute in Miami, ranked #1 by *U.S. News & World Report*. After several years at Washington Eye, he now heads The Zatezalo Group, a combined oculofacial plastics and ophthalmology center. He is affiliated with The Center for Facial Recovery, sits on the board of The Foundation for Facial Recovery, and serves as a consultant for the Sanctuary Cosmetic Center.

His scope of practice includes facial cosmetic surgery, including facial rejuvenation; revisional surgeries; browplasty (forehead lift); blepharoplasty (lid lift); periocular cancers and reconstructions; tear drainage disorders; lid abnormalities and orbital oncology; inflammatory disorders; and anophthalmic sockets. Dr. Zatezalo also specializes in nonsurgical facial rejuvenation using neurotoxins such as Botox® and Dysport® and dermal fillers such as JuvéDerm® and Restylane®, and scar revisions.

The Foundation for Facial Recovery extends special thanks to:

Christine Daly, SPT, Stockton University
Linda Johnson, Garden Gate Farm
Bonnie Lessans
Luis Miranda, Practice Manager, The Center for Facial Recovery
Stockton University
Andy Sussman
Juliana Wynkoop, SPT, Stockton University
Alison Winfield, Patient Navigator, Medstar Georgetown University Hospital, Department of
    Otolaryngology/Head and Neck Surgery

WHAT ON EARTH IS HAPPENING TO ME?

CHAPTER 1
Onset, Diagnosis, and Medical Intervention

Michael J. Reilly, MD

_____

"I woke up one morning with my eye burning and watering like crazy. When I was brushing my teeth and spit, the toothpaste went directly left. I looked up in the mirror and said, 'Oh, my God, I've had a stroke.'" —Dianna

Maybe you were putting on lipstick when you noticed your mouth seemed crooked. Maybe you were drinking a glass of wine when it inexplicably spilled down your shirt. Maybe you were arguing a case in court when your speech started to slur.

Wherever you were when you first realized something strange was going on with your face, you no doubt experienced the same moment of panic that grips nearly everyone whose face suddenly seems to go haywire: *am I having a stroke?*

Looking in the mirror, you might not have recognized half of your face.

Your smile was likely lopsided, with one corner of your mouth oddly drooping or unable to open. Your eye on the same side may have been unable to shut. Your brow likely refused to move. And your cheek was probably slack.

As the hours or days unfolded, a host of other symptoms may have unfolded, too, including:

- an intense headache
- pain on your face, in the back of your head, and especially behind and/or in your ear
- a red, swollen outer ear
- an intolerance for everyday noise levels, possibly accompanied by ringing of the ear or hearing loss
- vertigo or dizziness
- excessive drooling or a dry mouth
- copious tears or a dry eye
- less ability to taste or a metallic taste in your mouth
- frequent, accidental biting of your inner cheek and lip

This is the typical, harsh introduction to sudden facial paralysis.

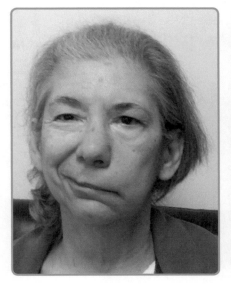 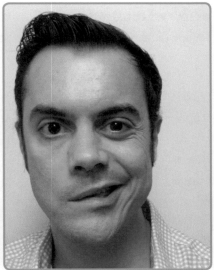 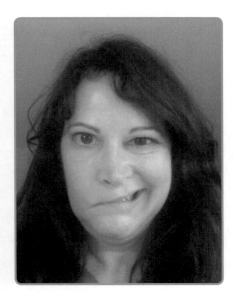

Three early-stage facial palsy patients showing the hallmark signs of the condition. Left and middle photographs courtesy of The Center for Facial Recovery. Photograph at right courtesy of the patient.

Tests to Expect

The doctor you see in a hospital emergency department, urgent-care center, primary care practice, or other healthcare setting will indeed first look for evidence of a cerebrovascular event (stroke), which can cause one-sided facial paralysis.

Hearing that a stroke has been ruled out will of course be a huge relief.

What happens next when you're being diagnosed can depend on whether your medical provider takes a conservative or aggressive approach to evaluating your case.

Every medical provider should ask about your health history and perform a thorough physical and neurological exam, paying close attention to how much loss of function there is in your face. If nothing concerning turns up and there is no likely explanation for your muscle weakness or paralysis, your doctor may determine you have **Bell's palsy, an inflammation of the seventh cranial nerve (also called the facial nerve).** Chapter 4 provides detailed information about this nerve and the surrounding facial anatomy.

Bell's palsy accounts for the majority of all sudden facial palsy cases. Because it's so likely, your doctor may not feel a need to conduct further tests. Other doctors may want to run additional diagnostics to rule out any underlying problem and check the amount of muscle activity. These procedures include:

- blood test or possibly a spinal tap to evaluate for Lyme disease
- blood test to evaluate for Ramsay Hunt syndrome (see page 6 for more on RHS)

- electromyogram (EMG) to assess the nerves that serve the muscles of your face. EMG can detect even minute movement in muscles, so it's an excellent diagnostic tool for people who seem to have complete paralysis. (Any bit of movement is good news!)
- computed tomography (CT) scan or magnetic resonance imaging (MRI) to rule out tumors or other problems

It's worth noting that absent any specific cause for concern, the benefit of administering MRIs in the early stages of facial palsy is not conclusive. Many experts find it more useful for someone whose symptoms have persisted for longer than two months. This caveat, coupled with the high incidence of cases turning out to be "just" Bell's palsy, may spur a patient to consider whether the expense is worth incurring.

So, You Have Your Diagnosis

What exactly is Bell's palsy? Named after Sir Charles Bell (1774–1842), the Scottish surgeon and anatomical artist who first documented the condition, Bell's palsy results when something causes trauma to, and swelling of, the seventh cranial nerve. This nerve is command central for the movement of your facial muscles. You have one on each side of your head. Chapter 4 illustrates and clarifies this further.

Briefly, the seventh cranial nerve, or facial nerve, emerges from your brainstem, runs through a long, bony canal under your ear toward your cheek, and then splits into five main branches. The trunk of the nerve is housed snugly inside the protective canal. It's a tight fit to begin with, and when an outside force agitates it, the nerve swells and then gets compressed by the canal. This prevents it from sending chemical messages necessary for movement in your facial muscles, causing weakness or paralysis and the symptoms you are now experiencing.

Recovery Rates

The most comforting news you will hear is that the majority of people with Bell's palsy will recover completely without any intervention. By the one-year mark, 71 percent are fully back to normal. Of those, most are recovered in three to six months; some even heal within a week or two.

The remaining people aren't so fortunate.

- Thirteen percent have a slight but permanent residual weakness.
- Sixteen percent have fair to poor recovery or never heal.

Researchers haven't been able to pinpoint why some patients recover and some do not. But they do know that a more difficult journey to healing is more likely for patients who:

- suffer prolonged, severe pain when symptoms develop.
- experience complete paralysis at onset versus mild paralysis or muscle weakness.
- haven't seen signs of recovery within six weeks.
- are older than age 60.
- are pregnant, diabetic, or have high blood pressure.

Estimates vary widely, but roughly 7 percent of people will experience a second attack of sudden facial palsy, perhaps years down the road, either on the same or opposite side of the face.

Symptoms show up and unfold within hours or over several days, almost always on just one side of your face. (Less than 2 percent of cases are bilateral, occurring on both sides.)

Bell's palsy strikes people of all ages, socioeconomic backgrounds, and gender. Even babies can get it, although it is most prevalent in people between the ages of 20 and 40.

Estimates vary, but in general, sudden facial palsy is thought to occur in more than 40,000 people each year in the United States alone.

Besides "How do I make this go away?", your number one question may be, "Why on earth did this happen?"

Causes of Facial Palsy

If you've been told you have Bell's palsy, it means that the exact cause can't be pinpointed. The case is considered idiopathic, which means "of unknown origin."

Much of the medical community, however, links most sudden facial palsy to a reactivation of the viruses behind cold sores (herpes simplex 1 virus), and chicken pox and shingles (varicella-zoster virus), which lay dormant in the body of people who've had any of those ailments. What resuscitates those viruses in the first place? Stress is a suspect, along with some correlated preexisting conditions:

- diabetes
- high blood pressure
- pregnancy (Pregnant women are 30 percent more likely to develop Bell's palsy—typically in the third trimester or shortly after birth—than women who are not pregnant.)
- lupus
- thyroid conditions
- sarcoidosis
- Sjogren's syndrome

In addition, dozens of other factors are thought to be capable of triggering inflammation in the seventh cranial nerve and thus facial palsy, including:

Other viral triggers

- infectious mononucleosis ("mono," or Epstein-Barr)
- respiratory illnesses (adenovirus)
- flu (influenza B)
- German measles (rubella)
- mumps (mumps virus)
- hand-foot-and-mouth disease (coxsackievirus)
- cytomegalovirus
- HIV/AIDS

Acquired conditions

- Lyme disease
- infections, including otitis media (ear infection)
- acoustic neuromas, cysts, and tumors near the facial nerve
- blunt-force trauma or injury to the face
- surgical wounds

Ramsay Hunt Syndrome: Facial Palsy, but Not Bell's Palsy

With its characteristic one-sided facial droop, asymmetric smile, and eyelid that can't close, Bell's palsy isn't hard to diagnose.

That's not necessarily the case for its potentially more serious "cousin," Ramsay Hunt syndrome (RHS). This is the second most common cause of sudden facial palsy and is known to be caused by the varicella-zoster (shingles) virus, or VZV. Simply put, Ramsay Hunt syndrome is a shingles attack on the facial nerve.

While Bell's palsy and RHS can mirror each other in symptoms, Ramsay Hunt syndrome can manifest with these tell-tale complications:

- extreme pain in or around the ear or in the face, head, or neck, often occurring after onset of facial weakness
- a rash or blisters, called herpetiform vesicles, in the inner ear or on the outer surface (and sometimes on the face, tongue, palate, larynx, and/or neck; the vesicles are sometimes overlooked, difficult to spot, or show up days after the onset of facial paralysis)

Additional symptoms may include:

- tinnitus (ringing in the ear), sensitivity to sound, and hearing loss
- vertigo, dizziness, and balance issues (sometimes leading to nausea and vomiting)

Differentiation gets tricky from there, however. Bell's palsy can *also* cause ear and face pain (albeit generally not severe), problems with hearing, and dizziness.

But the most complicating factor to getting a proper diagnosis of Ramsay Hunt syndrome is that often, the condition shows up with no blisters at all. **This form is called zoster sine herpete.** (Sine is pronounced SEE-neh.) **It may account for about one-third of cases initially thought to be Bell's palsy.**

Tests called serological or polymerase chain reaction assays can detect VZV antibodies or VZV DNA in skin and blood cells, saliva, or middle ear fluid, but it's not standard practice to run these tests.

Why is it so important to know if your facial palsy is Bell's or RHS?

Spontaneous recovery from Ramsay Hunt syndrome is far less likely than from Bell's palsy. Signs of recovery take longer to show up. And the treatment journey can be much more challenging as well.

However, rates of recovery are higher for people whose RHS is correctly diagnosed and treated early with a combination of steroids, antiviral agents, and therapy interventions.

_____

If you haven't started to recover within three months,
your condition is probably not Bell's palsy.

_____

Read on for more about managing the onset of sudden facial palsy with medication, regardless of what kind of facial palsy it is.

Get Those Meds!

The most important step you can take at onset is to begin a course of steroid and antiviral medication, ***ideally within 72 hours of onset.*** This is our belief based on some compelling research and on our clinical observations. In addition, there is mounting evidence for favorable outcomes when calcium channel blockers are used to treat patients with nerve weakness following trauma.

Here's what you need to know about these important drugs.

Steroid treatment. There are no magic bullets for treating sudden facial palsy, but treatment with systemic steroids appears to be the biggest game-changer. Numerous studies have shown improved recovery rates with the use of oral steroids, which act by decreasing inflammation in and around the facial nerve. These benefits have been shown to be greatest when the medication is started within the first three days. Although treatment with systemic steroid medication is not without potential adverse effects, we strongly believe that every consideration should be given to the use of this medication if at all reasonable based on your overall medical condition. If you are not prescribed a steroid by the initial provider you see for your facial palsy, we would highly advise that you seek a second medical opinion immediately to ensure this is in your best interest.

The vast majority of studies proving the effectiveness of steroid medication in the treatment of sudden facial palsy have used a dosage regimen of 10 days, typically beginning at a dose of 60 mg of prednisone daily for 5 days and then tapering off by 10 mg per day over at least 5 more days. However, the nerve inflammation that occurs from herpes simplex virus reactivation can persist for up to 3 weeks (based on the time required to completely heal oral ulcers) and the nerve inflammation from herpes zoster virus reactivation can persist for 4 weeks or longer (based on the typical duration of the skin rash that occurs with shingles). Because the exact cause of sudden facial palsy is not obvious in most patients, it is our recommendation to proceed with a 22-day treatment of steroid medication for all patients with complete paralysis if not medically contraindicated. This is an even stronger recommendation when treating patients with obvious Ramsay Hunt syndrome (shingles infection of the facial nerve). We begin with 60 mg of prednisone daily for 7 days, and then taper by 10 mg every 3 days over the next 15 days. For patients with facial pain symptoms indicating persistent viral neuritis beyond 3 weeks, we will strongly consider treating with additional steroids until the pain has resolved.

Unfortunately, the prescription practices for first-line providers treating facial paralysis vary widely. Some patients are given a much lower dose and shorter course than the 10-day course that has been studied in these large cohorts, and very few patients are treated with systemic steroid medication for a full 3 weeks. It is our hope that with increased awareness of this condition and its underlying biological causes, more providers will be willing to prescribe a longer duration of steroid medication for patients who are able to tolerate the treatment.

There are some special considerations regarding systemic steroids:

People with diabetes are at increased risk of developing sudden facial palsy and of having more difficult recoveries than people without diabetes. Yet many are treated with lower than recommended dosages of steroids due to concerns about the spike in blood glucose levels that may occur with such treatment. If you are diabetic, we highly recommend working with your provider to manage your blood glucose levels adequately with insulin or other interventions to ensure that you can still get on the necessary high-dose steroid regimen noted above if at all possible.

Women who are pregnant or nursing should check with their OB/GYN prior to starting steroids.

Antiviral medication. As we noted earlier, the two most common causes of sudden facial palsy are both viruses: herpes simplex (the strain that causes cold sores) and herpes zoster (the strain behind chicken pox and shingles and the known cause of Ramsay Hunt syndrome). Since antiviral medication is used to treat other herpes-caused illnesses like cold sores, chickenpox, and shingles, many physicians prescribe it for sudden facial palsy as well. A standard prescription would be a 7- to 10-day course of famciclovir (500 mg, 3 times daily), valacyclovir (1,000 mg, 3 times daily), or acyclovir (800 mg, 5 times daily).

It is important for us to be clear about the fact that much of the existing research on the use of antiviral medication for sudden facial palsy does not show a significant benefit. However, the two large clinical trials that came to this conclusion both evaluated the use of antiviral treatment for a total of *one week only*. We believe this to be an inadequate duration of treatment for determining the benefits of antiviral medication for the following reasons:

1. Vaccination studies have shown that the body's peak response to a herpes virus infection is typically around six weeks. After this, the battle between the body and the virus can ensue for months.
2. Only about 15 percent of patients with sudden facial palsy will show blisters or vesicles that are a clear sign of Ramsey Hunt syndrome, but molecular studies of the blood and saliva from patients with sudden facial palsy have shown signs of herpes zoster virus reactivation in approximately 39 percent of patients with sudden facial palsy.
3. Evidence has emerged in the past two decades that a prolonged course (12 months) of antiviral medication can help reduce the risk of damage from herpes virus-associated neural inflammation in the eye. The first study to show this benefit, called the Herpes Eye Disease Study, or HEDS,

was published in 1998 and showed a 45 percent reduction in long-term consequences of herpes simplex infection of the eye. Due to the positive findings from this study, a similar study, called the Zoster Eye Disease Study, or ZEDS, is now looking at the effects of prolonged antiviral treatment for herpes zoster (shingles) infection of the eyes. This is currently underway at the National Eye Institute, a division of the National Institutes of Health.

4. From studies of patients with shingles throughout the body, antiviral medication dramatically reduces the incidence and severity of long-term nerve complications. **It follows that the same reduction in long-term consequences from this virus could be expected with antiviral treatment for reactivations of the herpes zoster virus in the facial nerve.**

5. Patients with herpes zoster have been shown to have a 30 percent greater risk of stroke, and that risk appears higher when cranial nerves are affected. Thus, robust antiviral therapy may be prudent for herpes zoster-induced facial palsy in an effort to prevent an even more severe condition.

6. Finally, we have observed better clinical outcomes in our patients with severe cases of Ramsay Hunt syndrome who were given a prolonged course of antiviral medication for at least six weeks after onset of the condition.

As always when deciding whether to undergo a treatment, you should incorporate a thoughtful analysis of the risks and benefits. For facial palsy patients, there is a relatively high risk of incomplete recovery (25 to 30 percent). This alone would be enough to prompt consideration of anything that may offer some benefit.

When taken in conjunction with the very safe side-effect profile of the oral antiviral medications and the promising findings related to the use of antiviral medications in the management of other herpes-related nerve disease, we do recommend it to our patients.

———————

In addition, it is our hope that healthcare providers will not only consider early and prolonged (at least six weeks) antiviral medication for the treatment of sudden facial palsy, but that we can prompt enough consideration of this treatment rationale to foster future scientific studies. We believe these studies will ultimately prove the benefits of treating with a prolonged course of antiviral medications when confronted with sudden facial palsy.

———————

Calcium channel blockers. Recent literature has suggested the potential benefits of adding a calcium channel blocker to the medical regimen for the treatment of facial nerve weakness from injury (Lin et al, 2019) (Sin et al, 2018) (Tang et al, 2015). Calcium channel blockers have been used for years to dilate blood vessels in the treatment of hypertension. About 15 years ago, investigators began looking at the possibility of using these medications in the management of nerve dysfunction.

A recent meta-analysis (a review and statistical comparison of all relevant studies on a particular subject) indicated a 2.8 fold (280 percent) increase in the likelihood of complete facial nerve recovery after paralysis resulting from surgical or other traumatic injury to the nerve (Lin et al, 2019). The same study included outcomes for the use of calcium channel blockers in the treatment of vocal cord nerve paralysis resulting from surgical or traumatic injury to that nerve. For those patients, there was more than a 13-fold increase in the likelihood of complete recovery.

The theory is that calcium channel blockers work to help restore nerve function by promoting the growth of new nerve cells while also helping to prevent the death of existing nerve cells.

Based on this data, we have begun offering calcium channel blocker therapy to our sudden facial palsy patients, with frank discussion that this is neither current standard of care nor FDA-approved. While the side effect profile for calcium channel blockers remains fairly mild, there are adverse reactions. The greatest potential is for dizziness and/or lightheadedness due to a decrease in blood pressure. For this reason, we believe it is important for patients to monitor their blood pressure with a home blood pressure cuff and to make sure not to drive or perform any strenuous physical activity for at least a week after starting the medication.

Dosages in the above-referenced trials vary, but a regimen of 60 mg 4 times per day is a regimen that most patients can tolerate.

See page 11 for photographs of a preteen patient who received calcium channel blockers as part of his therapy regimen two months after the onset of his facial palsy.

Now that you understand what has happened to you and perhaps why, you'll need to smartly manage the day-to-day challenges of facial palsy that you are experiencing. See Chapter 3, Managing Day to Day.

CHAPTER 2
Facial Palsy in Children

Richard Redett, MD

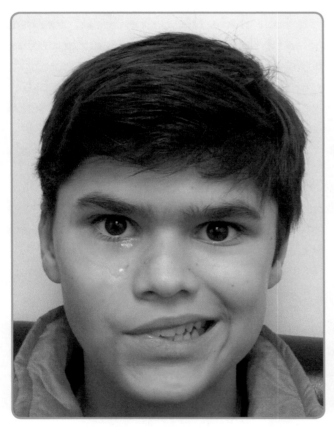

A preteen patient with Ramsay Hunt syndrome displays minimal smile function two months after the onset of his facial palsy. Photograph courtesy of The Center for Facial Recovery.

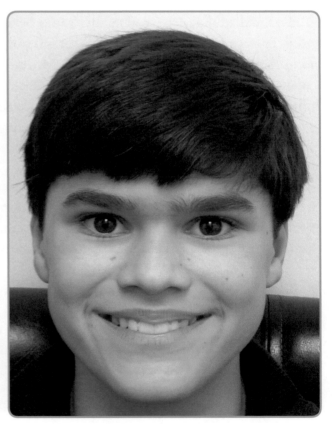

Significant smile improvement after 10 weeks of treatment. The patient had received steroid, antiviral, and calcium channel blocker therapy while undergoing facial rehabilitation physical therapy. Photograph courtesy of The Center for Facial Recovery.

Facial paralysis in young children can be as distressing for them and their parents as it is for adults who develop the condition. But tender-age patients have a big advantage: they tend to recover sooner and more fully than older people, either naturally or after surgery.

The condition can be either developmental/congenital (present at birth) or acquired (triggered by an external factor such as a virus or injury). Both kinds are relatively uncommon.

Congenital or Developmental Paralysis

As inexplicably as Bell's palsy strikes adults, facial palsy can also happen in utero for reasons that can't be explained. Babies who are otherwise healthy can emerge at birth with paralysis on one or both sides of their face. If no other anomalies are evident, their case is termed "isolated." If the paralysis is related to birth trauma, it will sometimes heal on its own.

A different kind of facial paralysis in newborns is **Moebius syndrome**, a rare congenital developmental disorder, characterized by the absence or underdevelopment of the nerves that control facial movements (cranial nerve seven) and eye movements (cranial nerve six). Most people with Moebius syndrome have weakness or complete paralysis of the facial muscles.

Children and adults with facial paralysis may be unable to smile, frown, raise their eyebrows, close their eyelids, or pucker their lips. This not only results in lack of facial expression but may also result in drooling and difficulty with speech. Children with Moebius syndrome also have motor delays due to upper body weakness, dry eyes and irritability, dental problems, cleft palate, and hand and feet problems, including club foot and missing or fused fingers. Moebius syndrome is always present at birth and is usually bilateral (involves both sides of the face). Other types of congenital facial paralysis usually involve only one side of the face. Although its origin is not well understood, it is thought to have a genetic or environmental link.

Because the condition is so rare—just 2 to 20 cases per million births—and the demands of their medical care are so extensive, the Moebius Syndrome Foundation (www.moebiussyndrome.org) was formed to create an in-person and online community of support for the whole family. A multidisciplinary team approach through a craniofacial center is often the most effective way to treat Moebius syndrome.

Acquired Facial Paralysis

Infection is the most frequent cause of acquired facial paralysis in children, and acute otitis media (the achy middle-ear infection that plagues so many babies and juveniles) is behind the majority of infection-generated cases. Other infectious agents include the herpes simplex virus, Epstein-Barr virus, cytomegalovirus, mumps, and rubella.

When facial paralysis is idiopathic, meaning doctors have no likely explanation for why it happened, it is called Bell's palsy.

Benign or malignant tumors, also called neoplasms, can paralyze the face. The facial nerve can also be damaged during surgery to remove them.

The last category of acquired paralysis is injury to the face. Examples of how this can happen include facial nerve-damaging accidents such as contact with a flying ball on the playground and, in babies, a forceps-assisted or otherwise difficult extraction at birth.

Fortunately, most cases of injury-acquired facial paralysis in both babies and juveniles heal quite well.

When Intervention Is Needed

All children who experience facial paralysis would do well to immediately be seen and then followed by a surgeon specializing in facial palsy to make sure they are progressing in a timely manner and without complications. Parents may be directed to consult with other physicians such as a pediatrician, neurologist, ophthalmologist, physical therapist, and maxillofacial surgeon. For school-age children, slow or nonexistent improvement in facial movement can be more easily addressed in the first nine months after onset; after that time, muscles can begin to atrophy or lose their tone, requiring more complex intervention.

Sometimes, children with facial paralysis don't or can't heal on their own. If their condition makes it difficult or even impossible to smile and form other expressions that convey emotion, or even eat and speak clearly, they can face devastating social challenges that may impact their self-esteem and quality of life. This can also be the case for affected adults, of course, but frequent social distress during the formative years can be especially fraught.

For this reason, medical professionals may suggest surgical procedures that can, in some cases, restore or create the ability to smile and interact more easily with other people. See Chapter 6 for more about these procedures.

It's important to note that surgical procedures for facial paralysis come with some caveats:

- Generally, the child needs to be older than age four.
- Every case is different, and the exact nature of the child's condition must be such that surgery is possible.
- Both the child and the family must be motivated after the surgery (and sometimes beforehand) to work, often for many months, with a physical therapist who understands facial palsy and can help the process of neuromuscular reeducation, which is training to optimize how the brain and muscles perform together.

CHAPTER 3

Managing Day to Day

Jodi M. Barth, PT, CCI / Lauren M. Bolding, DDS
Carl Chua, PT, CCI / Gincy L. Stezar, PTA, CCI

---

*"You don't really appreciate what your face does until
it doesn't do what it's supposed to do." —Tara, facial palsy patient*

So, a doctor has confirmed you haven't had a stroke—you've got facial palsy.

Hopefully, you've been given the recommended prescription for steroids. As we covered in the first chapter, studies have confidently shown that steroids taken within 72 hours of onset may shorten the duration and lessen the severity of your condition. Also, even though the effectiveness of antiviral medication is still being debated, we do recommend it in conjunction with steroids. (See page 8 for more on this important topic.)

Now it's time to take a deep breath and come up with a plan for dealing with the most pressing symptoms.

Seek Expert Guidance

Don't go it alone with sudden facial palsy, even if your recovery starts to happen rather quickly. Specialists from the following fields who have experience treating facial paralysis can optimize your recovery.

ENTs and Neurologists

These medical doctors specialize in disorders that impact the ears, nose, and throat areas and/or the neurological system. Those well versed in the treatment of facial palsy can counsel you on the pros and cons of various medications that can be helpful in the management of facial paralysis symptoms as well as recommend diagnostics to determine your proper course of care.

Ophthalmologists

These physicians focus exclusively on the prevention, diagnosis, and treatment of eye conditions and vision issues that can be associated with facial nerve palsy.

Oculoplastic Surgeons

Oculoplastics is a subspecialty of ophthalmology. When the function of the facial nerve has not recovered, the affected eye's surface can be compromised since the eyelids likely are not fully closing with each blink. An oculoplastic specialist can suggest interventions to assist with closure, improve tear drainage, address asymmetry, and more.

Facial Plastic Surgeons

These professionals have an expertise in complex facial nerve reconstruction procedures. Through their extensive knowledge of cranial anatomy and the facial nerve, their techniques can help lessen tightness and discomfort, restore movement, create a smile, and improve symmetry and function.

Physical Therapists

Facial neuromuscular retraining physical therapists are healthcare professionals whose practice focuses on the diagnosis and treatment of individuals of all ages who suffer from facial nerve-related conditions. All physical therapist are movement experts who optimize quality of life through prescribed exercise, hands-on care, and patient education. Rehabilitation of the face requires an expertise that differs from typical physical therapy intervention. It requires a thorough understanding of the distinct anatomy associated with the facial nerve and its muscles.

Occupational Therapists, Speech Therapists

These healthcare practitioners can also be facial nerve specialists whose focus is on the neuro-reeducation and functional restoration of the facial muscles. Their services include comprehensive evaluation, guidance, and education for those who suffer from facial palsy.

Dentists

Oral health professionals play an important part in managing facial palsy since diminished function of the mouth and tongue can contribute to oral disease. In addition to cavities and gum problems, these experts can address symptoms such as dry mouth, drooling, and facial pain.

Eye Care

In the first days, weeks, or months battling the complications of facial palsy, nothing requires more meticulous and persistent attention than taking care of your affected eye. As long as the eyelid can't completely close—a condition many Bell's palsy patients experience, called **lagophthalmos**—the eyeball is defenseless against injury and damage.

Chapter 5 discusses at length how facial palsy affects the eye at onset and when the condition persists long-term; the best ways to protect and comfort the delicate cornea; and the surgical procedures that can correct both functional and aesthetic complications. The most important things you need to know and do now bear repeating here.

Without a properly functioning eyelid, debris and dust can land on and injure the cornea. The cornea is the clear outer surface that protects the colored iris and much of the white part, too. It also aids with focus.

In addition, severe dryness can set in when lids aren't able to blink and spread the lacrimal gland's lubricating tears across the eye. Dryness is highly uncomfortable (contact lens wearers may need to switch to glasses), can trigger light sensitivity, and can cause blurry vision. Worse, dry eyes are at risk for infection, corneal ulcers, and even permanent loss of vision.

Here's what your eye needs right now.

Lubrication

You'll want to buy several packages of lubricating eye drops (*only* the preservative-free kind!) and keep some in your purse or pocket, in the car, by the TV, on your nightstand, and in the bathroom medicine cabinet. Note: Drops made with preservatives can sting, and people with severely dry eyes may develop preservative sensitivity or toxicity that makes symptoms worse. Plus, they can only be used a few times per day; you'll want relief more often than that.

Over-the-counter eye lubricants are available as eye drops (for daytime), gel drops (a thicker liquid for severe dryness), and ointment (a dense, greasy coating for overnight relief).

Simply using eyedrops alone may not be enough to stave off dry eye. Use drugstore eye ointment and a moisture chamber to maximize lubrication and form a physical shield against particles and drying elements at the same time. A moisture chamber is like a standard eye patch except it has a clear plastic "window" in the middle and spongey raised edges. Several kinds of moisture chambers can be found online. Your ophthalmologist or other physician may have suggestions for creating your own, too.

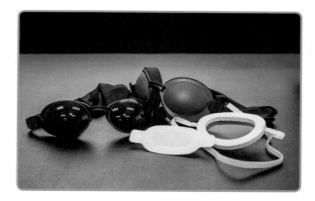

Moisture chambers to protect and relieve dryness in the eye. Clockwise from left: EyeEco's Tranquil Eyes goggles, EyeEco's Onyix Hydration Sleep Mask, Good-Lite Company's Moisture Chamber Patch, KLZ Medical's EyeLocc Eyelid Occlusion Dressing. Photograph by Andy Sussman.

Use Caution

Cloth eye patches can be helpful during the day, but they can scratch the cornea if the material accidentally touches the eye. This risk is greatest while sleeping and is one reason moisture chambers are better.

Many people try to protect their eye by taping the eyelids shut. There are safety concerns with this method, too. Never use cellophane tape—chemicals in the adhesive may irritate the thin skin around the eye. Surgical tape is better, as is hair-styling tape, but both kinds can pull out eyelashes and risk injuring the cornea if one of the edges nicks the eye during application or removal. If you must use tape, never adhere it vertically.

Sunglasses, especially the wraparound style, can protect the eye from sun sensitivity and the drying effect of the wind. Regular glasses with plain, no-prescription lenses (called "plano") are another choice for guarding the eye from the elements.

Do This Now!

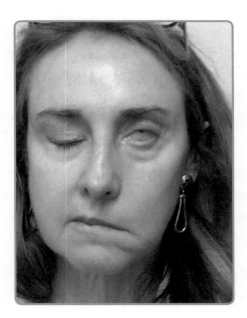

A facial palsy patient with lagophthalmos (incomplete eye closure) revealing the Bell's phenomenon. Photograph courtesy of The Center for Facial Recovery.

Our research indicates that the sooner eye closure returns, the less chance synkinesis (an extremely difficult complication to overcome) will develop.

Right now, though, your eye closure is likely being hampered by a normal process called the Bell's reflex, or Bell's phenomenon. This is a useful mechanism found in about 80 percent of people that causes the eyeball to roll up and to the side in a protective maneuver during a blink. But the strength of this reflex also makes eye closure harder, especially when your orbicularis oculi, a circular muscle around the eye area, is weakened by facial palsy.

To counter this, here's an exercise to start right away:

- Close your eyes.
- Take a selfie or ask someone to confirm that your affected eye is not completely shutting. This is an important step since it may not feel to you like your affected eye is open! (If your eye is still able to close—while sitting *and* lying down—you can skip this exercise.)
- Do the following sequence three times a day until your eye has recovered:

    a. Place your finger under your eye.
    b. Look down at your finger.
    c. Gently close both eyes and hold for a count of 10.
    d. Repeat 5 to 10 times.

Also see the eye-closure exercises on page 70.

Pain Remedies

Headaches and ear, face, and neck pain plague many acute facial palsy sufferers. Nonsteroidal anti-inflammatory drugs such as aspirin, ibuprofen, and naproxen may help, but if you were given steroids when you were diagnosed and are still taking them, be sure to clear any NSAIDs with your doctor first. They are contraindicated in combination with steroids. Gabapentin is sometimes used in adults to treat neuropathic (nerve) pain caused by the herpes virus or shingles (herpes zoster).

If you are medication-averse or are still having pain even with over-the-counter painkillers, you can add warm compresses or microwave beanbags to your regimen. Also worth trying are hand-warmer packs (the kind meant to be tucked inside gloves when it's cold out) placed where the pain is and then held in position with a scarf wrapped around your head. (If the pack is too hot, put a layer of the scarf or a piece of thin fabric between the pack and your face.)

In a similar vein, you may develop auditory hyperacuity—extreme sensitivity to noise that would otherwise be uneventful. Activities such as playing music, going to a movie, and eating in a restaurant may be intolerable. To help you cope, try removing yourself from difficult situations or using a pair of earplugs or musician-quality, high-fidelity headphones.

Breathing

An injured seventh cranial nerve can affect the sinus passages, in some cases leading to obstructed breathing and congestion that can be particularly bothersome at night.

Applying a breathing-assistance nasal strip at bedtime may help. Worn on the outside of the nose above the nostrils, these strips lift the sides of the nose to open nasal passages.

Eating and Drinking

As you've probably discovered, eating and drinking can be more than a little challenging with facial palsy.

An injured seventh cranial nerve hinders salivary/parotid glands, whose job it is to secrete fluid that eases the path of food down the throat. Luckily, in unilateral cases, the glands on the unaffected side will still produce saliva. Drinking plenty of liquids during meals should help compensate and minimize the risk of choking. Adding gravies and sauces to moisten your food can also help.

Whatever you eat, get in the habit of taking multiple napkins before you sit down to your meal. It's harder to keep food in your mouth when you have facial palsy, and because your tongue is probably less adept now at pushing food as you chew, you may need to manually help things along.

Drinking, whether from a glass or bottle, may also require special effort. In this case, try pushing up with your finger on the affected corner of your mouth to help your lips form a seal against the glass, or holding a napkin or cloth to your chin as you sip to catch any liquid that spills out.

Try experimenting with different kinds of glasses and mugs to see if one is easier to use—a coffee cup with a plain rather than curled rim, perhaps, or a lidded cup with a small opening that directs liquid into the middle of your mouth. Some people find that thin china cups are easier to use than thicker ceramic or glass vessels.

There are special cups on the market that are lightweight, semiflexible, and have a lower profile on one side to give the nose a wide berth and eliminate the need to tilt your head while drinking. The design also guides liquid right into the mouth.

Some people have an easier time drinking through a straw than with a glass and so carry a reusable straw with them when they're on the go. Others find it difficult to form a lip seal with a straw. Here, too, pressing up with a finger on the affected corner of the mouth can help. So can biting down on the straw as you sip.

Dental Care

You'll need a smart oral health regimen to protect vulnerable teeth and gums as soon as facial paralysis or weakness sets in.

Unaddressed, palsy can cause:

Tooth decay and gum disease. Cavities and inflamed or bleeding gums can be painful and are more likely to develop when these conditions are experienced:

- The mouth may not open fully, making it more difficult to brush and floss the side and back teeth. Child-size toothbrushes (or the smaller head on an electric toothbrush) can access difficult-to-reach areas. Likewise, floss holders (they look like tiny vegetable peelers) can navigate small mouth openings better than your fingers.

- Cheek muscles have a harder time retaining toothpaste or "swishing" plaque-fighting mouthwash (indeed, many people report that spilling or dribbling was the first sign that something was "wrong" with their face).
- A weakened tongue has a harder time clearing food particles from between the teeth and gums. This prolongs contact between protective tooth enamel and the corrosive sugars found in many kinds of food. If you can't brush your teeth after a meal, at least rinse your mouth well with water to prevent food from clinging to teeth.

It's a good idea to visit the dentist more frequently for professional cleanings. A dentist can also prescribe fluoride toothpaste and mouth rinses that have higher fluoride levels than drugstore products. These are generally used at nighttime, when the mouth is driest, to lay down an extra layer of fluoride on the teeth. The fluoride gels are sometimes applied via custom-made trays.

Dry mouth. Cavities (as well as bad breath) are also likelier if xerostomia, or dry mouth, sets in. It's the job of the parotid gland, and to a lesser extent the sublingual (under the tongue) and submandibular (under the jaw) glands, to produce saliva; it's saliva's job to keep cavity-causing plaque from forming and adhering to enamel. But these glands can become sluggish or nonfunctioning when palsy strikes, creating a drier environment that is a breeding ground for plaque and bacteria.

Signs of dry mouth include a sticky or dry feeling on the tongue, which can also interfere with clear speech; sores and mouth ulcers; taste disturbances; and a burning sensation.

Ask your dentist if taking medication to stimulate salivary flow is recommended.

Drooling. Some patients still produce adequate saliva but can't contain it. This isn't a medical concern but can be socially distressing. There are medications that can reduce saliva production, but not everyone is a candidate for it based on their existing medications and medical conditions. In addition, while the medication lessens the secretions of salivary glands, it also works in other areas of the body and can lead to unintended consequences.

Mouth sores. Eating with utensils and chewing food when half of the face isn't functioning properly inevitably results in painful bites to the lip or inside of the cheek. When an area is bitten, it swells slightly, leaving the area at greater risk for repeated biting or frictional irritation that can soon lead to sores.

For these wounds, dentists can prescribe a topical ointment to relieve discomfort while the sore heals. In some cases where a drooping lower lip continually gets caught in the teeth, a dentist may suggest taking an impression of the mouth to create a custom appliance that acts as a bite guard. Speak to your dentist to see if you are a candidate for this device.

TMD (Temporomandibular Joint Disorder). Some long-term facial palsy patients develop this painful condition of the jaw from chewing exclusively on the nonaffected side and throwing the muscles out of balance. The result can be constant or intermittent pain along with a clicking sound, or head and neck pain. A prosthodontist can diagnose TMD and suggest treatment, as can a physical therapist with experience treating facial palsy and TMD.

Denture Fit Changes. Because their cheek has lost tone, some facial palsy patients with false teeth find that their dentures don't fit as well. If they can wait several months to see if they regain muscle function, there may be no need to replace the appliance. But if a year has passed with no improvement, or if they are unable to tolerate wearing their prosthesis, they should discuss the situation with their dental specialist.

Proceed with Caution!

The urge to try anything to make your face better is understandable. But certain "remedies" have the potential to make matters worse.

Electrostimulation sends electrical current to muscles and nerve endings via electrodes placed on the skin. The therapy triggers muscles to contract and relax. This strengthens them, improves blood flow, and reduces pain. This has long been used on large muscles, ***but it is not able to precisely target smaller muscles like those found in the face.*** As a result, when used on facial palsy patients, the current also hits healthy muscle. In addition, when affected nerves begin to recover naturally, muscle tone starts to return—but adding additional current overstimulates the nerves and may disrupt nerve regeneration, as several studies in animals suggest. It can also lead to tight muscles and potential spasms. We believe this therapy may actually hasten or worsen existing synkinesis. The one exception is for patients who have prolonged (over a year) complete paralysis with no ultrasound-detectable muscle movement. Even then, the therapy should only be administered by an expert in facial palsy physical therapy.

Chewing gum. Some doctors tell their facial palsy patients to chew gum or otherwise rigorously exercise their facial muscles. However, this requires the activation of gross motor activity which can contribute to or worsen synkinesis, a devastating complication that causes parts of the face to move unintentionally when other parts are engaged.

Worth a Try

You likely will come across accounts from people who report that vitamin B-12 supplements, cannabidiol oil (CBD oil), and acupuncture helped them recover. When you hear praise for these measures, keep in mind that roughly 70 percent of people will recover from Bell's palsy without any treatment. That said, some evidence does point to their potential.

Can dental work cause Bell's palsy?

It's unsettling to contemplate, but at least one reputable study found a correlation between dental procedures and the onset of facial nerve palsy.

Cold sore eruptions, caused by the herpes simplex virus (HSV-1), have long been reported after dental work. HSV-1 in turn has been linked to the onset of Bell's palsy.

In the *Journal of Cranio-Maxillofacial Surgery* (January 2017), researchers reported that of nearly 2,500 patients, 16 developed facial palsy—14 with Bell's palsy, two with Ramsay Hunt syndrome—within an average of 3.9 days. The paralysis struck the same side of the face as where the procedure was performed.

The authors concluded that dental procedures were related to viral reactivation. They also found that the prognosis appeared worse for these patients than for people who develop Bell's palsy spontaneously.

Vitamin B complex and vitamin B-12 are well established as essential components for maintaining normal nerve function. So taking these as supplements for facial palsy would seem to have logical underpinnings. At least a few studies have shown a slight positive effect of these vitamins on accelerating nerve regeneration in laboratory rats. One of them compared B-12 to the supplement alpha lipoic acid and found positive evidence for both, with alpha lipoic acid having a slight edge. But studies examining the efficacy of vitamin B-12 supplements in treating facial palsy in humans are lacking.

Before trying these supplements, talk to your doctor about dosage, absorption issues, and medication interactions. Also discuss the pros and cons of taking methylcobalamin versus cyanocobalamin—two forms of B-12—and taking a tablet that you swallow versus a sublingual (under the tongue) product.

Consumer interest has intensified over **CBD oil**, or cannabidiol, which is derived from the Cannabis sativa plant (marijuana or hemp). Anecdotal evidence of the product's efficacy for easing pain and anxiety—common symptoms among facial palsy patients—has increased significantly, and some doctors even prescribe it for certain conditions.

Finally, acupuncture may well help with pain, tension, and anxiety. See Chapter 10 for more on this popular treatment.

Other Recommendations

Rest! Facial palsy can be mentally and physically taxing. Many people with the condition say they were tired or fatigued for weeks and even months after onset. Prioritize letting your body recuperate so it can expend energy on healing itself. This may mean taking time off from work.

Exercise. Although rest is important, regular aerobic exercise promotes increased circulation, produces endorphins (the body's natural pain suppressant), and can improve overall mental health. Let your body be your guide as to what you need and when.

Eat healthy. Despite what you may hear, there is no specific food or food combination that will "cure" facial palsy; likewise, there are no "bad" foods that will make your symptoms worse. (Too much added sugar can cause increased chronic inflammation, however.) Remember, your body functions best, and is most capable of fighting infections and injuries, when it's nourished with foods that are rich in protein, fiber, vitamins, and minerals derived from fruits, vegetables, legumes, whole grains, and lean meats.

Protect your face from the cold and wind to prevent your facial muscles from stiffening. Wrap your face in a scarf when outside so your breath can warm your cheeks. Avoid sitting or sleeping under air conditioners or ceiling fans.

Find your tribe. No one can understand what you are experiencing better than other people with facial palsy. Online support groups welcome newcomers and are a rich source of empathy, humor, commiseration, coping strategies, self-care tips, and more. Facebook, for example, has several groups, including one strictly for "long-timers." To start, search the site for the keywords "Bell's palsy," "facial palsy," "Ramsay Hunt syndrome," and "acoustic neuroma."

As with anything you read online from nonmedical sources, be sure to vet any health and therapy information with your healthcare provider before trying something, since group members sometimes share detrimental advice. Touting chewing gum as an effective muscle activator is just one example.

And take with a grain of salt someone's claim that supplements, dietary modifications, essential oils, or any other single factor was responsible for their quick recovery: remember, the majority of people with Bell's palsy recover on their own.

Document your progress with dated selfies, videos, and journaling. It may become important, for example, to know how long it was before movement started to return, or where exactly you experienced pain. The history can also be a big morale booster when you look back and see how far you've come.

Speaking of morale, read about coping emotionally when your condition does not resolve in Chapter 11.

Of course, in addition to managing your symptoms, you're probably eager to explore ways to start healing. But first, see the next chapter to gain a deeper understanding of your facial anatomy, which will benefit your recovery efforts.

Facial Paralysis Care Kit

- Pain remedies:
  - warm compress
  - microwavable beanbag
  - heating pad
  - over-the-counter nonsteroidal anti-inflammatory drugs, such as aspirin, ibuprofen, and naproxen (NSAIDs) or acetaminophen (do not take NSAIDs without a doctor's clearance if you are taking steroid medication)
  - scarf and hand-warming packs
- Eye care:
  - preservative-free eyedrops
  - lubricating eye gel and ointment
  - moisture chamber (commercial)
  - sunglasses, especially wraparounds
  - no-prescription ("plano lens") glasses
- Oral care:
  - drinking straws
  - therapeutic cup with one side cut lower
  - oral irrigator
  - flossing sticks/picks
- Earplugs or musician-quality, high-fidelity headphones
- Massage oil or lotion
- Nasal strips

CHAPTER 4

Anatomy and Trauma of the Seventh Cranial Nerve

Kalpesh Vakharia, MD

The seventh cranial nerve, also called the facial nerve, controls the vitally important mimetic muscles that generate facial expression. These muscles convey our emotions and help us communicate with other people. This is one reason why seventh cranial nerve injury can be so traumatic for people with facial palsy.

Facial muscles are unique in that they are the only muscles in the body that have voluntary or controlled activity (e.g., you smile when thanking someone) and involuntary activity (your brow furrows when you're angry).

They are also distinctive because most of them insert into skin or fascia rather than bone. Which means that whatever is happening to the skin directly impacts the muscles' ability to function. Small and delicate, the facial muscles are susceptible to contracture, tension, deformity, and weakness. And, because facial nerve trauma mostly affects one side of the face, when afflicted they can create an asymmetrical appearance with the unaffected side.

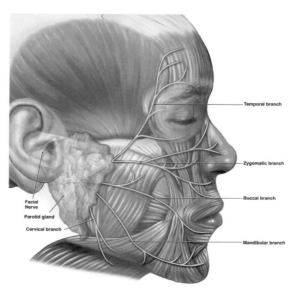

Path of the seventh cranial nerve and its five main branches. Illustration by DIOMEDIA/Nucleus Medical Media.

In addition to governing facial muscles, the seventh cranial nerve is also responsible for

- some of the muscles that assist with swallowing.
- the lacrimal, or tear-producing gland.
- the salivary, or saliva-producing glands.
- two-thirds of the tongue's role in taste.
- sensation of the ear.
- the stapedius muscle of the middle ear, which protects it from excessive vibrations.

Until now, your seventh cranial nerve was able to send a vital, movement-triggering signal from the brainstem to the facial muscles.

But now, something has triggered inflammation in the nerve on one side of your face and caused it to swell inside the narrow, bony canal encasing it. (Chapter 1 discusses the many factors thought to be capable of disrupting the seventh cranial nerve.)

This compression interferes with the nerve's job, which is to deliver chemical agents called neurotransmitters to the muscles to power them to move. When the nerve is inflamed and swollen, the chemical response that these muscles need to activate is not received. Muscle activity is weakened or halted, producing the facial paralysis, asymmetrical features, and functional problems you are experiencing now. (If both sides of your face are affected, you have bilateral facial palsy; this happens in less than 2 percent of cases.)

The Nerve's Path

It's easy to imagine the seventh cranial nerve, which is one of 12 to originate in the brainstem. It runs in front of and below your ear, cuts through your parotid gland, and then tracks over the side of your face before splitting into five main branches. These branches send electrical impulses to the facial muscles from the forehead to the neck. To visualize where they reside, place the base of your palm underneath your ear and let your fingers fall loosely across your face. The five branches roughly correspond to where your fingers rest.

These branches of the seventh cranial nerve are called, from top to bottom:

- **temporal** (or frontal) branch, controlling muscles of the forehead and eye
- **zygomatic** branch, controlling eye and cheek muscles
- **buccal** branch, controlling muscles between the eye and the corner of the mouth
- **mandibular** branch, governing the lower portion of the mouth
- **cervical** branch, controlling the neck's platysma muscle

Smaller nerves shoot off from these branches as well, each connecting to very specific areas of muscle.[1]

---

[1]   This is why we do not advise electrostimulation, which broadly distributes current.

Muscles Behind the Trauma

The following is an overview of what happens to the various facial muscles when the seventh cranial nerve and its branches are traumatized. Note that some muscles receive directions from more than one branch, while some branches govern more than one muscle.

It may be helpful to refer back to this section during treatment as needed.

MUSCLES OF THE HEAD

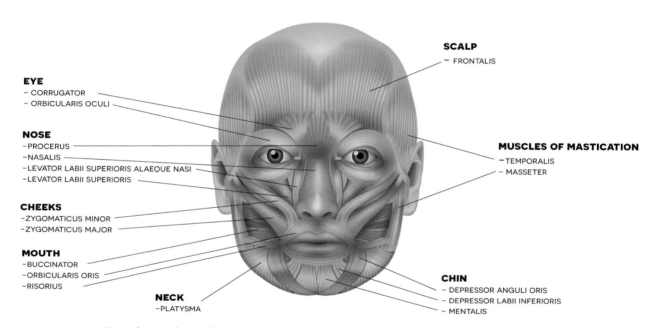

Facial muscles and the areas they govern. Illustration by Tefi / Shutterstock.

Your smile is distorted, with one corner drooping.

- Nerve branches: zygomatic, buccal, and mandibular
- Muscles: zygomaticus major, zygomaticus minor, levator anguli oris, levator labii superioris, orbicularis oculi, risorius, depressor anguli oris, and depressor labii inferioris.

Your cheek has gone slack, has no tone, and looks "melted."

- Nerve branches: zygomatic and buccal
- Muscles: zygomaticus major and minor

Your lips will not pucker.

- Nerve branch: buccal
- Muscles: orbicularis oris and buccinator

Your eyelid cannot close or only closes partway.

- Nerve branch: temporal
- Muscles: orbicularis oculi and corrugator supercilii

You can't raise your eyebrow or furrow your brow.

- Nerve branch: temporal
- Muscles: frontalis, corrugator, and procerus

You can't wrinkle your nose.

- Nerve branches: temporal and buccal
- Muscles: corrugator supercilii, nasalis, depressor septi nasii, levator labii superioris, and aleque nasii

Forehead and eye wrinkles disappear—but only on the affected side.

- Nerve branch: temporal
- Muscles: frontalis, corrugator, and orbicularis oculi

You have "oral disability," or a hard time working your mouth properly. Tongue and lip impairment cause drooling and slurred speech when pronouncing b's, p's, and s's (consonants that require lip seal). Food and drink spill from your mouth. You accidentally bite the inside of your lip and cheek.

- Nerve branches: marginal mandibular, buccal, and zygomatic
- Muscles: orbicularis oris, buccinator, upper lip levator, lower lip depressor, zygomatic major, and risorius

Your sense of taste on your tongue is diminished, or you notice a metallic taste.

- Nerve branch: the chorda tympani, which is a branch of the facial nerve that relays sensations of taste from the front part of the tongue and runs through the middle ear. This branch of the facial nerve exits the ear and joins the lingual nerve.

You have pain in front of or behind the ear; you develop noise sensitivity, ringing in the ear, hearing loss, and/or dizziness.

- In severe attacks, other cranial nerves besides the seventh or facial nerve may be affected, especially the trigeminal nerve and the vestibulochochlear nerve. The trigeminal nerve is cranial nerve five and sits close to the facial nerve in the brainstem. Because it is responsible for sensation to the face, when it is not working, you might feel pain or numbness. The vestibulocochlear nerve, cranial nerve eight, also is close to the facial nerve. It is responsible for balance and hearing. Damage to this nerve could cause stability issues, dizziness, and changes in hearing.

Now that you know where your symptoms originated, you'll be better able to understand the mechanisms behind the many complications that can develop, and how healthcare professionals with experience treating facial palsy can partner with you—and each other—to improve your recovery.

I JUST WANT THIS
TO GO AWAY!

CHAPTER 5

Facial Nerve Palsy and the Eye

Chad Zatezalo, MD

"When I could close my eye again, it was exhilarating!" — _Sharon_

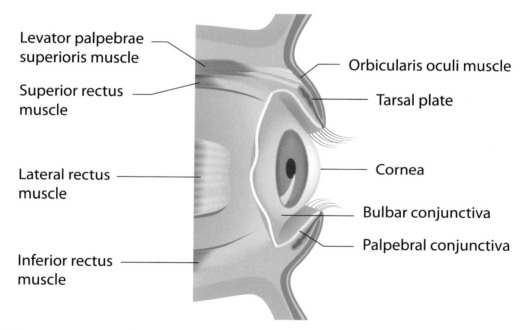

Facial palsy patients must take care to protect their cornea, the clear outer surface that covers the eye in front of the colored part, called the iris. Illustration by Alila Medical Media / Shutterstock.

Seventh nerve palsies, including Bell's palsy, can trigger numerous short-term and long-term complications.

It is imperative to get a proper workup to determine the correct diagnosis as management and treatment are based on your condition. Not all patients will receive the same treatment since not all facial nerve palsy cases are Bell's palsy. Regardless of the diagnosis, anyone experiencing an inability to blink should consult with an ophthalmologist or oculoplastic surgeon. An oculoplastic surgeon is a sub-specialized ophthalmologist who has the highest level of training in eyelids, orbital tissue (eyeball, eye muscles, optic nerve, and bones around the eye) and the tear drainage system.

A complete workup will examine the ocular surface, eyelid tone, and a factor called blink dynamics. Blink dynamics refers to how the nerve disruption in facial palsy can impair the speed of voluntary and involuntary blinks; when the eyelids do not blink efficiently, the surface of the eye can be compromised. Fluorescein (a special dye) may be used to better visualize the ocular surface. After the exam, the physician will review the treatment options and recommendations.

Understanding the Blink

There are two main surfaces of the eyeball: the cornea and the conjunctiva (see image at left). The cornea is the clear outer surface of the eye in front of the iris and the pupil. The conjunctiva is the clear lining in front of the sclera, the white component of the eye.

When the eyelids function appropriately, the upper and lower lid touch with every blink and completely cover the cornea and conjunctiva. This action both protects the vulnerable eyeball and distributes a tear film over the surface to keep it lubricated. However, in facial nerve palsy, the nerve is unable to sufficiently carry a signal that normally tells the lids to move. This insufficient signal leads to an incomplete blink, also known as **lagophthalmos**, and may result in a host of secondary symptoms that include but are not limited to redness, irritation, burning, blurry vision, infection, ulceration, tearing, and loss of vision. These occur from a lack of vital tear film that the entire ocular surface depends on the eyelids to deliver.

Tears: More than Water

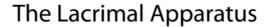

The Lacrimal Apparatus

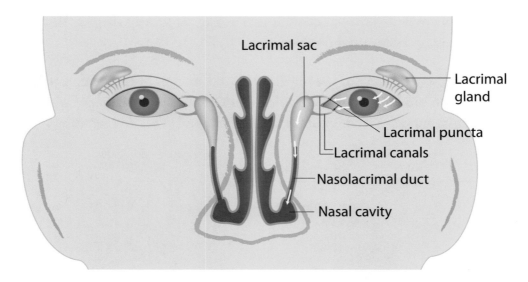

Lacrimal gland and tear-drainage anatomy. Illustration by Alila Medical Media / Shutterstock.

The tear film is made of three layers: mucous, water, and oil (see page 32). Mucous is made by the cells on the eyeball, water by the lacrimal gland (located just above the eyeball), and oil by the glands within the eyelids. The oil prevents evaporation of the water within the tear. Each eyelid houses approximately 30 oil glands, also referred to as **meibomian glands**. With each full-strength blink, tension in the eyelid increases and expresses oil from each gland. However, when poor blink function reduces this tension, the oil stagnates. Stagnant oil can lead to inflammation of the eyelids and ultimately result in a chalazion, also known as a sty.

Stagnant oil also leads to evaporative dry eye. People with lagophthalmos can ward off evaporative dry eye by applying warm compresses, which will decrease the viscosity of the oil. (Think olive oil versus toothpaste.) Decreased oil viscosity makes it easier for the oil to be expressed, even with compromised eyelid tension.

Other variables may affect how well an eye is able to tolerate an inefficient blink. Patients who, prior to getting facial palsy, had another medical condition that affects the ocular surface are more at risk for blink-related complications. They should make sure their prior condition is optimally addressed and then discussed with an ophthalmologist.

Diagnoses affecting the ocular surface include but are not limited to diabetes, thyroid-related diseases, rheumatoid arthritis, and other arthritis-related diseases. Certain classes of medications, including antidepressants, allergy and cold medicines, and blood pressure medications, can also affect the ocular surface and should be reported to your ophthalmologist.

Why A Dry Eye Tears

A common symptom associated with dry eye is tearing. When the ocular surface is compromised or unhealthy, the eye sends a message to the brain to produce more tears. In turn, the brain sends a signal to the lacrimal gland, the gland that produces the water component of the tear, to increase production. However, there is no corresponding increase in the mucus and oil components, which are responsible for holding the tears on the eyeball. Without enough mucus and oil to help them adhere, the excess tears overwhelm the tear drainage system and overflow.

Overflowing tears are also a product of the impaired blink function in facial nerve palsy. The pressure system generated by each blink is dampened, which retards active tear drainage. When both the blink dynamics and the ocular surface are compromised, the likelihood of tearing increases.

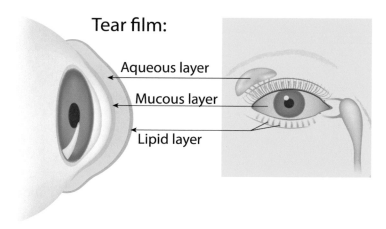

Layers of the tear film. Illustration by Alila Medical Media / Shutterstock.

It may seem counterintuitive, but adding additional, artificial tears can help with tearing due to dry eye disease in facial palsy. To understand this concept, think *quality* of the tears. In dry eye disease, the use of artificial tears decreases the concentration of inflammatory mediators which are harmful to the eye.

In facial nerve palsy, placement of an artificial tear treats the unhealthy surface of the cornea and conjunctiva by coating the ocular surface with a more viscous material than the native tear. Decreasing the surface area of the cornea/conjunctiva exposed to direct ambient air creates a better environment for cells to replicate, which improves the health of the ocular surface.

Medical Treatment Options (to be prescribed by your physician)

The following is an overview of some of the treatment options for facial nerve palsy. Creating a treatment plan is the art and science of being a doctor. Not every patient will benefit from each of these treatments, and some treatments may lead to additional damage in certain cases. This section is not a substitute for medical care and is not intended to guide your medical treatment, but only to act as a source of information.

Nonsurgical Treatments

Lubrication. Lubrication of the eye can lead to a healthier ocular surface and improve comfort levels. There are several preparations on the market to help with this: liquid drops called tears, gels, ointments, and oil-containing products. Depending on the severity of your condition, your doctor will suggest a regimen of one or a combination of these products. Some of the products contain preservatives that can be toxic to the cornea, especially when used excessively.

Protection. There are several ways to protect an eye with lagophthalmos from the environment.

- *Moisture chamber:* This is a commercially available device (see page 16 for examples) that lubricates as well as protects the eyeball. There are also several methods to create your own moisture chamber. Please consult with your physician for guidance.
- *Scleral contact lenses:* Custom-made for you, these are larger than regular contacts. They extend beyond your cornea onto the white part of your eye (the sclera) and provide moisture by creating a chamber of solution between the lens and the cornea.
- *Patch:* Some patients feel better even with a simple eye patch covering their affected eye as this minimizes contact between the ocular surface and the environment.

Surgical Interventions

Lid loading. Lid loading procedures increase the weight of the upper lid. With extra weight, less tension is required in the eyelid muscle to make it drop, so the blink is more efficient. Gold and titanium weights are the two most popular, but other metallic choices exist in myriad shapes and forms, including eyelid springs.

Your physician will determine if lid loading will help your condition and the most suitable kind of weight if so. He or she may also discuss nonsurgical methods to load the lid.

Tarsorrhaphy. There are several types of tarsorrhaphies, but each of them involves surgically adhering the upper and lower eyelid to decrease the surface area of the eye exposed to the environment. As with all surgical treatments, there are pros and cons to this option. The major downfall is the cosmetic outcome.

Punctal plugs. Typically made of silicone, punctal plugs are a medical device used to block the flow of tears in the tear drainage system. Plugs are usually used for patients who have extreme dry eye and minimal symptoms of tearing. Not every patient with a facial nerve palsy or Bell's palsy needs or should have punctal plugs.

If tearing ensues after a plug is placed and does not resolve over the first week, the plug is often removed.

Lateral canthal tendon and orbicularis tightening procedure. In Bell's palsy, a diminished signal from the seventh nerve can erode the static and dynamic tone of the upper and lower lids by weakening the circular orbicularis muscle. The orbicularis is a sphincter muscle whose normally static tone dynamically increases when contraction—i.e., a blink—occurs. But as the static tone of the orbicularis muscle decreases, the upper lid rises and the lower lid falls. This is known as eyelid retraction secondary to a decrease in orbicularis tone, a neurologic phenomenon.

The canthal tendon and orbicularis tightening procedure, which involves making a small incision through the skin where the upper and lower eyelid meet near the cheek, combats the decrease in static and dynamic tone. The results are less eyelid retraction and a more efficient blink. A more efficient blink in turn improves the health of the ocular surface and allows for better expression of oil from the Meibomian glands.

Lower lid retraction repair. As the tone of the orbicularis muscle decreases, the lower lid falls inferiorly (meets the eye at a lower point). Tightening of the lower lid alone may not adequately elevate the eyelid. In these cases, the lower lid can be raised using one of several techniques. The gold standard is placing a hard palate graft into the lower eyelid.

How it works: The lower lid has a muscle that raises the lid (orbicularis) and one that lowers the lid retractor. In Bell's palsy, the muscle that raises the eyelid does not work as well; the muscle that lowers the lid wins out, and a net lowering occurs. To alleviate this, the muscle that lowers the lid is released from its attachment point to the eyelid, and a piece of tissue from the roof of the mouth (the hard palate) is placed between the attachment point and the muscle. This allows for more complete coverage of the ocular surface and increases the chance that the eyelids will kiss on each blink.

Nonsurgical approaches can also elevate the lower lid but are more complex in nature and not performed by all surgeons.

Upper lid blepharoplasty and brow lift. With Bell's or another seventh nerve palsy, the brow often falls. The descent of the brow is referred to as brow ptosis. (Ptosis is used to describe a descent of most anatomical structures.) When the brow falls, the eyelid skin can appear redundant and interfere with the field of vision. In addition, the brow and forehead can often feel heavy if function of the forehead muscle does not recover. In these cases, surgical repair may be an option.

The upper face is a single unit with three components: brow height, skin redundancy, and eyelid height.

In order to rehabilitate the upper face, each component needs to be addressed and repaired if necessary. If one component is neglected, the result will be unsatisfactory.

Component 1: the brow

Lifting a brow in a patient with Bell's palsy or a seventh nerve palsy often increases facial symmetry and improves the superior and lateral visual fields. There are many techniques for elevating a brow and several for fixating it into position. The method a surgeon deems best for a patient will depend on factors such as hairline, gender, skin type, and severity of the brow ptosis.

Component 2: the upper eyelid skin

Usually when the brow has fallen, the upper eyelid skin appears redundant and folds on itself. If the ocular surface is healthy under microscopic evaluation and the patient is asymptomatic and not tearing, the patient may consider combining an upper lid blepharoplasty (eye lift) with the brow lift. This can be a high-risk surgery if the patient has a poor blink and an unhealthy ocular surface. If surgery is performed, care should be taken to only remove skin and leave the orbicularis uninterrupted. If the orbicularis is removed, the patient's blink and thus the ocular surface may worsen. On the other hand, if the patient has significant synkinesis, removing the orbicularis may be beneficial.

Component 3: eyelid height

An upper eyelid that appears to be drooping may in fact be the result of synkinesis. If this is the case, surgical elevation is not the preferred approach and treatment should focus on the synkinetic activity. There are multiple treatment modalities for synkinesis. Neurotoxins such as Botox™ and Dysport™ can provide a temporary fix. Surgical procedures that aim for more permanent improvement also exist.

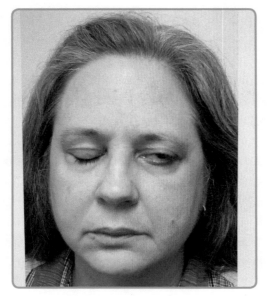

Patient presenting with lagophthalmos, an inability to fully close the eye. Photograph courtesy of The Center for Facial Recovery.

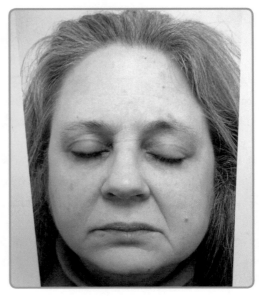

Patient after a lid-loading procedure. Photograph courtesy of The Center for Facial Recovery.

CHAPTER 6

Facial Restoration with Plastic Surgery

Christine M. Clark, MD / Michael J. Reilly, MD

"Right away [after surgery], the movement of my bottom lip was stronger. I'm getting more turn-up now. I didn't go into this feeling like I'd come out looking 'normal,' but every time I see family members, they say I look better and better. I feel normal. I feel confident. I would totally do this again."

—Nicole, Ramsay Hunt syndrome patient, three months after modified selective neurectomy to restore smile symmetry

---

"Synkinesis makes my eye shrivel like a raisin when I smile and eat; Botox® does wonders for this. I call it 'God's magic juice.'"

—Felicia, seven years with Ramsay Hunt syndrome

The good news for facial palsy patients is that experienced facial plastic surgeons can usually do something to benefit anyone with this condition. This is true regardless of whether the condition developed recently, has existed for many years, or was present at birth (called congenital facial palsy).

The caveat is that the cause of the paralysis, the extent and duration of symptoms, and numerous other variables (age, other medical problems) factor into the *level* of improvement patients can expect to see, as well as the treatment options that are suitable for them in the first place.

For those with sudden paralysis (usually from viral inflammation of the seventh cranial nerve), the duration of facial palsy and the probability of complete recovery are highly variable. However, there are some generalities to consider (see Table 1) (Marsk, et al 2012).

Table 1: Likelihood of Complete Recovery from Sudden Facial Paralysis

Duration/Severity of Sudden Paralysis	Likelihood of Complete Recovery
Incomplete (still some movement)	Nearly 100%
Signs of movement within 4 weeks	90%
Signs of movement within 6 weeks	85%
Signs of movement within 8 weeks	50%
No signs of movement by 12 weeks	< 5%

For those with incomplete paralysis (still some movement of the face even at its weakest point), complete recovery is almost always obtainable. If the facial movement begins to return within four weeks, then chances of complete recovery approach 90 percent. After four weeks, there is a gradual decrease in the rate of complete recovery. If there are no signs of recovery by 12 weeks, is very unlikely complete recovery will occur.

First Things First

While most patients will visit their primary care, prompt care, or emergency provider at the onset of facial palsy (see Chapter 1), we highly recommend follow-up with a facial nerve specialist as soon as possible, no later than two weeks from the onset. There are three aspects to this condition that are time-sensitive and warrant immediate consultation:

Measuring the degree of nerve signal disruption. Studies have shown that if more than 90 percent of the nerve signal is disrupted between three and 14 days after sudden paralysis as measured by a special electrical study on the facial muscles called an EMG (electromyogram), there is potential to improve recovery rates with an urgent surgical intervention (McAllister, et al 2013). In these circumstances, a procedure called nerve decompression may help if performed within the first three weeks (see page 45 for more about this, including risks). These nerve decompression surgeries are performed by a two-surgeon duo: 1) a highly specialized ear, nose, and throat physician called a neuro-otologist and 2) a neurosurgeon.

Ensuring adequate eye closure. An inability of the affected eyelid to completely close may leave the eye exposed and vulnerable to damage. Patients in this case should see an oculoplastic surgeon (eye specialist), facial plastic surgeon, or ophthalmologist. These specialists can educate patients on how to care for the eye themselves and in some cases may recommend a minimally invasive procedure to prevent serious damage and loss of vision. (See Chapter 5 for more on plastic surgery and the eye.) In addition, a physical therapist with experience treating facial palsy can work to loosen tissue surrounding the eye that may be restricting closure along with the underlying paralysis.

Ensuring an optimal medical regimen. Irreversible nerve damage may occur as early as three weeks from the onset of facial palsy. For this reason, it is imperative that patients in the narrow window after diagnosis are managed with the best possible medical regimen. Many first-line providers are not experts in the management of this condition and do not have a nuanced understanding of the potential for incomplete recovery. The general medical community believes sudden facial palsy to be a serious problem, but one that

THE FOUNDATION FOR FACIAL RECOVERY

"almost always" resolves completely with time. However, large studies have shown that approximately 25 percent of patients with sudden facial palsy will not fully recover (Engström, et al 2008). Thus, we see a critical need to optimize the medical regimen in these few precious weeks of care. Providers that are most likely best equipped to manage this condition include specialized ENT physicians called otologists, facial plastic surgeons, and neurologists with a special interest in facial palsy.

Talk to your provider about their familiarity and comfort level with treating your condition, including their knowledge about the chance of incomplete recovery. If your provider is not a self-identified expert in the condition, it is reasonable to ask at the very least for a prescription for a high-dose steroid taper and antiviral regimen (see Chapter 1). Then seek an immediate follow-up consultation with a facial nerve expert.

For those patients who do not have complete recovery from their facial paralysis by three months after onset of the condition, it is beneficial to consult with a facial plastic surgeon to discuss additional treatment options, including injectable treatments and surgery.

Nonsurgical Treatment

Chemodenervation (Botox® Injection) for Facial Spasm

Chemodenervation is a vital part of how many facial palsy patients manage their condition.

Bell's palsy patients whose nerve fibers regrow abnormally find themselves struggling with synkinesis (a form of a neurological disorder called hemifacial spasm). They endure the frustration of muscles on one side of their face involuntarily contracting, usually during times when attempting to move different facial muscles. This often causes uncontrollable facial distortion and uncomfortable tightness in the face and neck.

Chemical denervation (the use of an injectable medication to reduce nerve input to the wrong areas) can temporarily treat these symptoms. This procedure lessens undesirable muscle activity via injection of botulinum toxin (a bacterial toxin) directly into the affected areas. This treatment is commonly known by the brand names Botox®, Dysport®, and Xeomin®. (See page 43 for suggested guidelines for first-time patients.)

The effects of botulinum toxin can temporarily treat the symptoms, with the effect typically lasting about three months. It may diminish sooner or later than that average, however. While Botox® does not offer a permanent solution to the issue, regular treatment will often help quiet the undesirable nerve pathways that have formed after facial paralysis.

What Botox® Injections Entail

A small amount of Botox® is injected into each of the desired areas using a 30-gauge needle. Each injection will leave a pinpoint mark and a small lump from the fluid into which the Botox is mixed. The lump usually resolves in about 15 to 20 minutes.

Post-Procedure Recovery

Botox takes effect within three to seven days, at which point there should be less sensation of tightness and improved symmetry. Less than 5 percent of patients see mild bruising. Icing the area and applying a topical arnica gel or ointment can expedite healing.

What to Expect

Repeated Botox injections for issues related to facial paralysis are almost always covered by major insurance carriers. While there are general guidelines regarding dosages for the different facial areas, every patient is unique. Often, the minimum amount will be used the first time, since over-injecting and unintentionally weakening muscles is always a risk. It is important to work with your physician to generate an ideal treatment regimen for you as an individual. This may involve a follow-up visit after the medication has had time to take full effect so that adjustments to the dosages can be made if necessary. **Don't give up after the first treatment if you don't feel like it has delivered the desired effect. This is a highly personalized treatment that may require several sessions to tweak to an individual patient's needs.**

Overall, this treatment shows excellent promise for treating the discomfort and visible asymmetries associated with incomplete recovery of facial paralysis. It is most effectively done in tandem with physical therapy as part of a larger neuromuscular recovery plan.

The following patients demonstrate how beneficial botulinum toxin therapy can be for treating facial palsy.

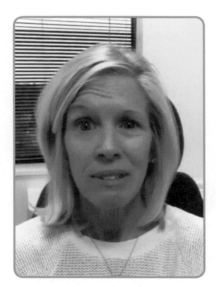

Patient A, who presented with left-side facial palsy and chronic hemifacial spasm, performs the "eyebrow raise" exercise. Note the limited upward mobility of the left brow, overcompensation of the right brow, exaggerated forehead lines, synkinesis of the eye, and chin dimpling.

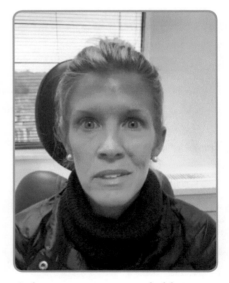

Patient A demonstrating remarkable improvement during a follow-up visit 21 days later. Symmetry is restored to the brows, eyes, and forehead while the chin is smoother. There are often some mild rejuvenating benefits as an ancillary benefit of this treatment. In this patient, the "crow's feet" have been softened in an effort to improve symmetry and reduce the undesirable synkinetic eye closure on the left (reader's right).

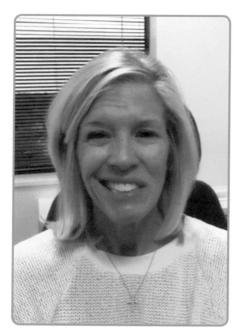

Patient A smiling before chemodenervation.

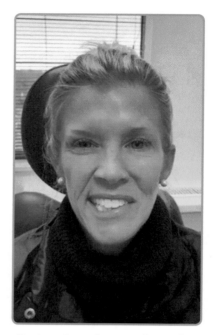

Patient A smiling 21 days after receiving 50 total units of Botox.

Patient A was injected on her left and right sides with 50 total units of Botox, with dosing as follows:

Right side (reader's left):

2.5 units into medial frontalis
2.5 units into central frontalis
1.25 units into lateral frontalis
5 units into lateral orbicular oculus
2.5 units into the inferolateral orbicular oculus
2.5 units into the zygomaticus major muscle medially

Left side (reader's right):

5 units into the lateral orbicularis oculus
1.25 units into the inferior orbicularis oculus
5 units into the mentalis
10 units into the medial platysmal band (5 superiorly, 5 inferiorly)
12.5 units into the lateral platysmal band (5 superiorly, 7.5 inferiorly)

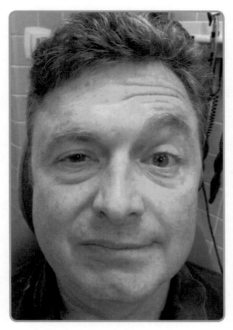

Patient B, who has right-side facial palsy, shows synkinesis and hemifacial spasm while attempted brow elevation prior to getting 70 units of Botox.

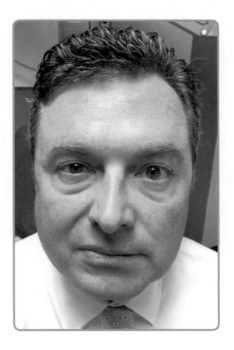

Patient B 33 days post-Botox injections.

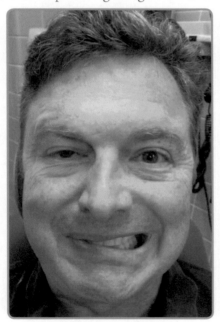

Patient B smiling before chemodenervation. Weakened and fibrotic smile muscles (zygomaticus major and minor) prevent the right corner of his mouth from turning up and spasming muscles cause significant squinting in the affected right eye.

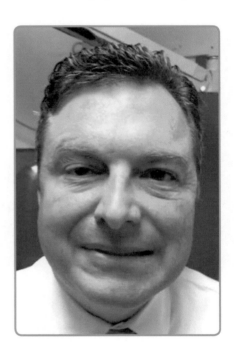

Patient B shown again smiling 33 days after receiving Botox therapy. All Botox patient photographs courtesy of Michael J. Reilly, MD.

Treatment for Patient B included the following injections:

Right side (reader's left):

5 units into the orbicularis oculus
5 units into the mentalis
25 units into the platysma (10 medially, 15 laterally)

Left side (reader's right):

5 units into the corrugator
12.5 units into the frontalis
7.5 units into the orbicularis oculus
5 units into the zygomaticus major muscle
5 units into the depressor angularis oris (2.5 inferiorly and 2.5 mid-belly)

Chemodenervation: A Suggested Approach to Botulinum Toxin Therapy for New Patients

The following are dose ranges based on our own experience of more than a decade performing chemodenervation for patients with facial spasm as the result of incomplete recovery of facial palsy. These guidelines incorporate countless conversations with patients, other facial palsy specialists, and a review of the academic literature on the subject (Bilyk, et al 2018). The goal of these treatments is to optimize facial harmony and symmetry by decreasing input to relatively overactive muscles in the unaffected side of the face and decreasing input to muscles that are either under too much tension and/or are causing undesirable movement in the affected side of the face.

The values presented here cover the vast majority of patients, though there are always exceptions. Having open communication with your doctor about your goals for treatment will be the best way to ensure an optimal result.

Note: For most patients, it requires at least three sessions of chemodenervation to determine the optimal dosing.

UNAFFECTED SIDE

Area/Function	Muscle Involved	Suggested Starting Dose
Forehead	Frontalis	2.5–15 U
Brow furrow	Corrugator	5–10 U
Crow's feet	Orbicularis oculus	2.5–12.5 U
Smile	Zygomaticus	2.5–5 U
Snarl	Levator labii nasii	2.5–5 U
Upper lip	Orbicularis oris	1.25–5 U
Lower lip	Orbicularis oris	1.25–5 U
Frown	Depressor angularis oris	2.5–5 U
Lip lowering	Depressor labii inferioris	1.25–2.5 U

AFFECTED SIDE

Area/Function	Muscle Involved	Suggested Starting Dose
Forehead	Frontalis	1.25–5 U
Brow furrow	Corrugator	2.5–10 U
Crow's feet	Orbicularis oculus	2.5–15 U
Under eye	Orbicularis oculus	1.25–5 U
Inner cheek	Buccinator	2.5–5 U
Frown	Depressor angularis oris	2.5–5 U
Neck	Platysma	5–30 U

Injectable Fillers. Various facial fillers can help balance asymmetries that occur as a result of facial paralysis. The most common filler material is hyaluronic acid, a gel-like synthetic material that is also naturally occurring in the human body. Popular products include Juvéderm®, Restylane®, and a host of others.

Physical Therapy (Neuromuscular Retraining). Neuromuscular reeducation is done to help "retrain" the brain, muscles, and nerves in a new way to optimize function. It is universally prescribed as part of the facial plastic surgeon's overall treatment plan, which may involve other interventions as well. This therapy is best performed by a physical therapist who has experience treating facial palsy (see Chapter 7).

Surgical Treatment

Surgical treatment is typically reserved for patients with chronic facial weakness (symptoms lasting more than 12 weeks). For these patients, there are numerous options available to significantly enhance quality of life.

Many patients who consult with a facial plastic surgeon do so in hopes of regaining facial symmetry—having a smile that appears more even on both sides, or an affected eye that looks roughly the same size as the other. Another frequent goal is getting relief from a constant, uncomfortable feeling of tightness or tension in the affected cheek and neck.

In the case of facial palsy, plastic surgery can help a patient look more like themselves and feel more comfortable, both physically and socially. Various procedures can

- restore the ability to express emotion.
- improve impaired speech.
- correct vision obstructed by a drooping eyelid.
- relieve chronic dry eye or excessive tearing.
- lessen or eliminate drooling and difficulty eating.
- alleviate anxiety and depression by correcting one or more of these complications, which frequently create major emotional, social, and professional challenges.

Know Before You Go

Plastic surgery for facial palsy requires careful evaluation by patient and physician alike. Here are some important considerations when deciding to pursue surgical treatment for facial paralysis.

Communication is Key. A good physician will assess (and continually reassess) a patient's goals and work with them accordingly. Not every patient has the same appetite for surgical intervention. Nor does every patient find that their asymmetry affects their self-esteem. Some may merely want to eliminate tightness and discomfort; others may only want to address their weakened eye but not their mouth, or vice versa.

Age Plays a Part. While younger people may have more noticeable gains with certain surgical interventions, older patients can also make impressive gains. The pros and cons of surgical treatment can be discussed with patients at any age.

Insurance May Help. People who pursue facial plastic surgery strictly for aesthetic reasons typically are denied coverage by health insurance plans. But because of the significant functional deficits that facial palsy can cause—difficulty speaking, eating, seeing, and sometimes hearing—many insurance plans will authorize full or partial coverage of surgeries and injectables. The physician's office will often assist with seeking preauthorization.

Every Case Is Different. It's a good idea to not form preconceived ideas of what's possible for you until your consultation. Your expectations may not be realistic; likewise, you may have more reason to be optimistic than you feel. Regardless, the statement that "results may vary" applies to all plastic surgery procedures—facial palsy or not.

It's Likely to Be an Ongoing Process. Many of the surgical treatment plans for issues related to facial palsy require two or more staged procedures. Due to the complexity of the condition, optimal effect may not be attained after a single surgical session. A good plastic surgeon should take a conservative approach that starts cautiously and proceeds after evaluating results.

As noted above, neuromuscular reeducation done by an experienced physical therapist will typically maximize the results of plastic surgery. Ideally, the therapist and surgeon will consult with each other over the course of the patient's care.

Surgical Procedures to Improve and Restore Facial Function

There is a wide variety of surgical procedures that can help restore facial movement. This section is meant to provide a broad overview of these procedures. The process of deciding which surgery is the best option is highly individualized and depends on many different factors, and your facial plastic surgeon is the best resource to determine which procedure(s) would be best for you based on your goals.

As noted at the start of this chapter, a procedure called **nerve decompression** can make a critical difference in the early stages (the first three weeks) of paralysis. Decompression of the facial nerve is a fairly invasive procedure and involves removal of bone around the narrowest region of the canal that houses the highly inflamed seventh cranial nerve (the facial nerve). Removal of this bone eases the pressure on the nerve and allows it to work again. It may sound like an easy choice, but it's a controversial procedure that comes with several caveats:

- It's only appropriate to consider in cases where the patient has an electromyogram (EMG) showing a near-complete paralysis of the facial nerve—at least 90 percent. An electrodiagnostic test is the only way to accurately assess the degree of nerve impairment, because patients may *appear* to have complete paralysis when in fact they do not.

- Beyond three weeks from onset, there is no demonstrated recovery benefit.
- It carries its own significant risks, including permanent hearing loss and permanent damage to the facial nerve. Many facial plastic surgeons will not perform nerve decompression because of these inherent risks.

After the initial three-week window, facial plastic surgeons have a host of other options to restore facial movement. These procedures fall under the umbrella term of **facial reanimation.**

The main factor that determines which facial reanimation procedure will work for a particular patient is the type of muscle impairment that is present: non-flaccid or flaccid.

Patients are considered to have **non-flaccid** palsy if they have some underlying nerve function, but that function is being waylaid by synkinesis and fibrosis. (See pages 56 and 57.) In patients who have had complete facial paralysis for a year or longer, the native muscles in the face irreversibly lose their function and become what is known as **flaccid**. Therefore, a new muscle must be used to restore the smile and movement in the lower face. There are more patients with non-flaccid palsy than flaccid palsy.

What follows is an overview of the facial reanimation procedures available for both categories of palsy.

Non-Flaccid Muscle Option

PROCEDURE: Modified Selective Neurectomy
(Also called selective neurolysis)

Suitable for: Facial palsy patients with some facial movement and synkinesis

Goals: Restore the smile's symmetry and spontaneity; alleviate tightness in the face and neck; improve the look of the mouth at rest; help the mouth to function better

Entails: Taking advantage of the beneficial nerve input still present by "rewiring" the nerves

Underneath the face near the ear, the surgeon uses electrodes to carefully identify which nerves are functioning properly and which ones have regenerated abnormally and are working against the smile. Nerves that help with showing the upper and lower teeth are preserved; the others are deactivated. Typically, one of the aberrant nerves is connected to a primary smile nerve to provide more power to the desired area. A *platysma myectomy* to release the pull of the platysma muscle in the neck is usually performed during this surgery as well.

Pros: The facial plastic surgeon who developed this procedure, Babak Azizzadeh, MD, reported outcomes for 63 patients who underwent modified selective neurectomies between 2013 and 2017. Most patients achieved significant improvement—some almost immediately, others over the course of several months—and none experienced long-term complications (Azizzadeh and Frisenda, 2018) (Azizzadeh, et al 2019).

An additional benefit of this procedure is a short recovery process. Patients typically go home the same day after surgery. And, should a patient experience another episode of Bell's palsy later, it's thought—but not proven—that the nerve "rewiring" from selective neurectomy will prevent a recurrence of synkinesis, but there would be no protection from the temporary muscle weakness or paralysis.

Cons: Selective neurectomy does not reduce synkinesis or asymmetry of the eye region, and about 20 percent of patients may require a second neurectomy to achieve optimal results. Lingering issues with weakness around the corner of the mouth may also be encountered, but the majority of these issues resolve within three months of surgery.

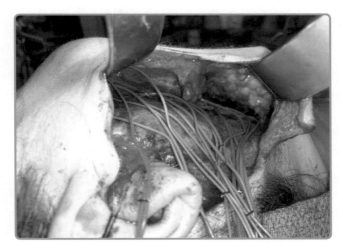

During selective neurectomy, dysfunctional nerve branches (tagged with blue markers) are intentionally cut; desirable nerves (tagged with red markers) are preserved. Photograph courtesy of Michael J. Reilly, MD.

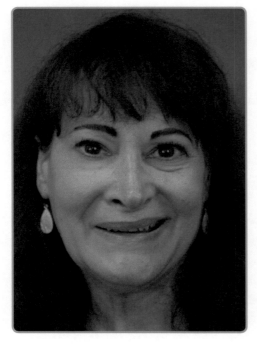

A patient with limited smile excursion due to synkinesis six years after acute facial palsy onset. Photograph courtesy of Michael J. Reilly, MD.

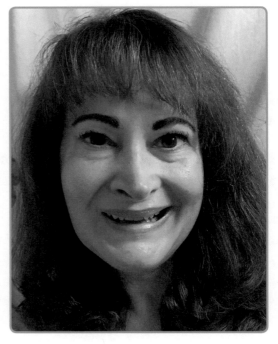

The patient three-and-a-half months after undergoing modified selective neurectomy. Photograph courtesy of the patient.

Flaccid Muscle Options

PROCEDURE: Static Tissue Repositioning

Suitable for: Patients with long-term facial paralysis (more than one to two years). After this time, the muscles in the face have lost their function.

Goals: Create better facial symmetry; address drooling, lip biting, and other side effects of paralysis

Entails: Lifting the corner of the mouth and the fold that runs between the corner of the mouth and the nose (laugh line) to an anchor point on the bone just below and behind the eye

This procedure is done with endoscopic equipment in order to minimize incision size. It is usually performed through a combination of a small incision in the laugh line and a small facelift incision behind the ear. The graft is then placed under the skin where it is not visible.

Patients can opt to use one of two materials to bridge the gap between the mouth and the anchor point: Alloderm or Tensor Fascia Lata.

Alloderm is freeze-dried, customizable cadaver tissue that is readily available and has been used for decades all over the human body. Alloderm tends to integrate well with the surrounding tissue and has a very low risk of rejection. **Tensor Fascia Lata** is strong connective tissue that the surgeon harvests from the thigh through a small incision. The advantage of Tensor Fascia Lata is that the material is taken from your own body, and this further lowers the risk of infection and/or rejection but does involve two surgical sites (face and thigh).

Pros: The effects are immediately seen once swelling from surgery subsides. This is different from other procedures such as the gracilis muscle transplant, where results take time.

Cons: No movement is restored to the face. The Alloderm and fascia can stretch with time, so the benefits are not permanent.

PROCEDURE: Muscle Transfer—Gracilis Muscle Transplant
(Also called free flap surgery or free tissue transfer)

Suitable for: Patients with long-term complete facial paralysis (more than one to two years), at which point the native facial muscles have lost their ability to regain function. Some surgeons are now offering this procedure for patients with non-flaccid paralysis but weak smile function.

Goal: Restore movement to the lower facial muscles and create a smile

Entails: Harvesting a piece of inner thigh muscle (gracilis muscle) for use in the face. Sometimes this requires two surgeries.

This procedure recreates facial function by using a working nerve from a different site to power the transplanted gracilis muscle. There are three nerves that are typically used to power the gracilis muscle: the working facial nerve on the other side of the face, the masseteric nerve, and the hypoglossal nerve. There are pros and cons to each of these nerves, and your surgeon will talk with you about which nerve option(s) would work well to help you achieve the best possible result based on your goals.

The surgery involves taking a small portion of the gracilis muscle, along with its artery, vein, and nerve (obturator nerve), which are removed from their locations at the inner thigh and connected to an artery and vein in the head and neck region using a highly specialized microsurgical technique. The connection of these blood vessels is critical for the muscle to survive in its new environment. The new nerve arrangement powers the gracilis muscle to move in a direction to simulate the natural smile muscles.

In 2016 in the *Journal of Cranio-Maxillofacial Surgery*, Dr. Bianchi published outcomes for 42 patients who had undergone gracilis muscle transplants powered by cross-facial nerve grafts in the *Journal of Cranio-Maxillofacial Surgery*. He found significant improvements in patients' quality of life and social functions. (Bianchi, et al 2016).

Here are more specifics on each of the three nerves that can be used to power the gracilis muscle:

Contralateral/Normal Facial Nerve Via Cross-Facial Nerve Graft

- *Nerves involved:* The facial nerve on the other side of the face, and the sural nerve, which is a sensory nerve from the lower leg.
- *Entails:* When this nerve is used, it often requires two surgeries. During the first surgery, the sural nerve is removed from the leg and attached to the facial nerve on the other side. The other end of this nerve is then tunneled under the skin to rest in the paralyzed side. Because this nerve graft crosses the face from the non-paralyzed side to the paralyzed side, it is called a cross-facial nerve graft. The second surgery is usually done six to nine months after the first surgery to allow time for the nerve signal to grow from the non-paralyzed side to the paralyzed side. During the second surgery, the cross-facial nerve graft is connected to the nerve that moves the gracilis muscle.
- *Pros:* Allows for a spontaneous smile without the need for deliberate movement such as jaw clenching (as with masseteric nerve transfer) or tongue protrusion (as with hypoglossal nerve transfer).
- *Cons:* Usually requires two surgeries, results in numbness of the fifth toe and side of the foot due to sural nerve harvesting, may result in a weaker outcome in older individuals.

Masseteric Nerve

- *Nerve's role:* This nerve helps move the masseter muscle, which helps you to chew.
- *Entails:* Rerouting one of the branches of the masseter nerve to power the gracilis muscle.
- *Pros:* The masseter nerve is strong and easily accessed during surgery.
- *Cons:* When this nerve is used, it requires teeth clenching to smile. Though this initially takes practice and exercise, smiling becomes effortless in the majority of patients over time. There is also a theoretical risk of trouble when chewing after this surgery, but the chance of this happening is low.

Hypoglossal Nerve

- *Nerve's role:* This nerve moves half of the tongue.
- *Entails:* Part of this nerve can be rerouted to power the gracilis muscle.
- *Pros:* The hypoglossal nerve is very strong and fairly easy to access.
- *Cons:* There is a small risk of tongue weakness that can lead to difficulties with speaking and eating. There is also a risk of inadvertent facial twitching when moving the tongue, such as during eating. Practice and exercise are required to help coordinate tongue movement for the smile.

PROCEDURE: Temporalis Tendon Transfer

Suitable for: Patients with long-term facial paralysis

Goal: Provide voluntary facial movement

Entails: Transferring one of the muscles used for chewing from the jawbone to the corner of the mouth

Temporalis tendon transfer is helpful for patients who are not candidates for more advanced facial reanimation procedures like cross-facial nerve grafts. This procedure is performed through small internal and external incisions between the nose and mouth, and it typically has very good results. The patient learns to move the face by contracting the relocated temporalis.

Pros: With dedicated exercises, patients can obtain voluntary control of the movement of the corner of the mouth, replicating a smile. Patient satisfaction following temporalis tendon transfer has been shown to be relatively high in several research papers. In a study published in *Archives of Facial Plastic Surgery* (2007), it earned a mean satisfaction score of 8.5 (from a possible score of 10) in patients who underwent this procedure. Another study published in *JAMA Otolaryngology–Head and Neck Surgery* (2018) compared outcomes in mouth symmetry and smile excursion for temporalis tendon transfer and gracilis muscle transplant. They found that both surgeries significantly improved mouth symmetry and smile excursion, though the improvement in smile excursion was higher in patients who had undergone gracilis muscle transplant. (Byrne, et al 2007) (Oyer, et al 2018).

Cons: The newly restored movement does require effort and is rarely spontaneous.

PROCEDURE: Nerve Graft—Masseteric Nerve

Suitable for: Patients with long-term facial paralysis

Goal: Increase control of the facial muscles

Entails: The masseteric nerve helps to move the masseter muscle, which helps you chew. This nerve can be connected to the facial nerve to help with facial movement. It can also be used to power the gracilis muscle during a gracilis muscle transplant (see gracilis muscle transplant above).

Pros: The masseter nerve is strong and easily accessed during surgery.

Cons: When this nerve is used, it requires teeth clenching to smile. Though this initially takes practice and exercise, smiling becomes effortless in the majority of patients over time. There is also a theoretical risk of trouble chewing after this surgery, but the chance of this happening is low. The recovery of facial tone at rest is usually apparent within six months. Older individuals may take longer to achieve the desired function, but the end result is usually comparable to younger individuals.

PROCEDURE: Nerve Graft—Hypoglossal Nerve

Suitable for: Patients with long-term facial paralysis

Goal: Increase control of the facial muscles

Entails: Connecting the hypoglossal nerve, which helps move half of the tongue, to the facial nerve to help with facial movement. It can also be used to power the gracilis muscle during a gracilis muscle transplant (see gracilis muscle transplant, above).

Pros: The hypoglossal nerve is very strong and fairly easy to access.

Cons: There is a small risk of tongue weakness that can lead to difficulties with speaking and eating. There is also risk of inadvertent facial twitching when moving the tongue, such as during eating. As with the masseteric nerve, practice and exercise are also required to help coordinate tongue movement for the smile.

PROCEDURE: Cross-Facial Nerve Graft

Goal: Restoring spontaneous facial movement

Suitable for: Patients with long-term facial paralysis

Entails: Harvesting a nerve from the lower leg, connecting it to a nerve in the unaffected side of the face, and then tunneling under the skin to connect to one of the facial nerve branches on the affected side.

When this nerve is used, it often requires two surgeries. During the first surgery, a nerve that is involved in sensation to the lower leg, called the sural nerve, is removed and attached to the facial nerve on the unaffected side. The other end of this nerve is then tunneled under the skin to rest in the paralyzed side. Because this nerve graft crosses the face from the non-paralyzed side to the paralyzed side, it is called a cross-facial nerve graft. The second surgery is usually done six to nine months after the first surgery to allow time for the nerve signal to grow from the non-paralyzed side to the paralyzed side. During the second surgery, the cross-facial nerve graft is connected to the nerve that moves the gracilis muscle.

Pros: Allows for a spontaneous smile without the need for deliberate movement such as jaw clenching (as with masseteric nerve transfer) or tongue protrusion (as with hypoglossal nerve transfer)

Cons: Usually requires two surgeries, results in numbness of the fifth toe and side of the foot due to harvesting the sural nerve and may result in a weaker outcome in older individuals.

Risks to Consider

All facial plastic surgery procedures involve a certain amount of risk and have limitations. Although the risks of facial reanimation procedures are relatively low, they do exist. Potential complications from surgery include and are not limited to bleeding, infection, pain, scarring, difficulty getting around (though it is rare for this to be a long-term problem), numbness, failure to improve, worsening of facial weakness and symmetry, and flap failure (death of the tissue or muscle that was transferred due to compromised blood supply).

The strength of and control over the reconstructed smile continues to improve over several years. Over time, the brain has the potential to undergo a reeducation process called cerebral adaptation that results in the production of a more naturally occurring smile even in cases where nerves other than the facial nerve were used to provide the input.

Vet Your Surgeon!

There are thousands of talented plastic surgeons in the United States alone who can spectacularly improve unaffected people's appearance with injectables and fillers, facelifts, brow lifts, blepharoplasty (eyelid and undereye surgery), and other common procedures. It's even becoming common to find general practitioners who offer botulinum toxin and other appearance-enhancing injectables.

But as you may have already discovered, the above-mentioned repertoire does not necessarily indicate a provider's ability to optimally treat your facial palsy. **The appropriate professional to treat you is, at a minimum, one who is highly specialized in plastic surgery of the face.**

The American Academy of Facial Plastic and Reconstructive Surgeons (AAFPRS) and the American Society of Plastic Surgeons have physician-finder tools on their websites (www.aafprs.com and www.plasticsurgery.org, respectively) that will help you locate a qualified professional in your area. Still, not every facial plastic surgeon is equipped to care for patients with facial paralysis. When consulting with a surgeon, be sure to ask these questions:

- **What board certifications do you hold?** Many states do not require a physician to have specific training in plastic surgery in order to perform cosmetic and reconstructive procedures.
    - In the U.S., for eyelid and other facial plastic surgical procedures, your physician should be board certified by the American Academy of Facial Plastic and Reconstructive Surgery, the American Board of Plastic Surgery, or hold a certification from the American Society of Ophthalmic Plastic and Reconstructive Surgeons.
    - For treatments related to the eye itself, your physician should be board certified by the American Board of Ophthalmology.
- **How/when/where did you train in the procedure I am considering?**

- **How many times have you performed this procedure in the past year, and what kind of results have you seen?** (It's just as important to talk about complications patients may have experienced as it is to talk about success stories).
- **How many facial palsy patients do you see in a typical month or year?** Even board-certified ENTs, ophthalmologists, and plastic surgeons who want to treat facial palsy have to start somewhere, so make sure you are comfortable with their expertise before proceeding with an intervention.
- **How often do you go to conferences focused on the treatment of facial paralysis?** When was the last time you read a peer-reviewed publication about facial paralysis?
- **What course of action would you recommend if your family member or close friend came to you with my same situation?** Are you confident in your ability with this, or would you refer me to another specialist who is more experienced?
- **May I see before-and-after photos of patients on whom you have performed the treatment we are discussing?** Ideally, the physician will have a "look book" or website with examples of their work. Ask if these photos showcase only their *best* outcomes, or if they also reflect *typical* results.

CHAPTER 7

Harnessing the Power of Physical Therapy

Jodi Barth, PT, CCI / Carl Chua, PT, CCI / Gincy Stezar, PTA, CCI

"Being proactive has provided me with some control over this complicated condition."
—Leah, Ramsay Hunt syndrome patient

Two schools of thought govern when to begin physical therapy treatment for facial palsy.

Some practitioners advocate waiting until a patient has gone three months with little or no recovery. Others find benefit in having a patient begin physical therapy immediately to receive in-depth education, guidance, and treatment.

Those of you who've just developed facial palsy may wonder: why start physical therapy if there's a chance I will be one of the roughly 70 percent of people who fully recovers?

Our clinical findings indicate early intervention promotes better outcomes for those who find themselves in the 30 percent of the facial palsy population with delayed healing and slow recovery. Since it's difficult to know at onset which category you will fall into, we believe seeing a facial palsy physical therapist early is the optimal approach.

And just as it's never too early, it's never too late to seek help.

Getting Started

Whether you've just developed facial palsy or have had it for a long time and are now seeking treatment, your first session should start with a comprehensive evaluation of your condition, including relevant health history.

The information presented in this book is not intended to replace professional diagnosis or treatment of any facial condition. Seek prompt medical attention for any sudden abnormal appearance or dysfunction of the face. Descriptions of physical therapy treatments, products, and suggested exercises are for informational purposes only unless discussed with or carried out by a qualified, licensed facial palsy therapist. See page ii for a full disclaimer.

Your therapist will ask you to perform a series of basic facial movements—and ideally, capture them on video and/or still photography. Using one of several universal grading scales, they will assign a number to indicate how much movement there is in each of the involved muscles. These numbers, as well as the videos and photographs, will be important for you and your therapist to measure your progress at subsequent visits.

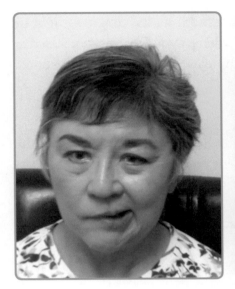 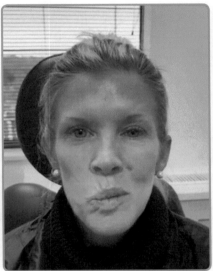 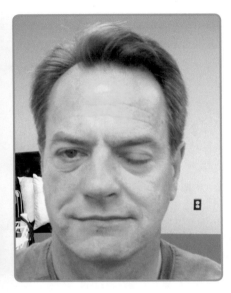

Patients with facial palsy demonstrate three of the facial movements used to assess degree of muscle movement. Left: A patient with Bell's palsy attempts an open-mouth smile. Photograph courtesy of The Center for Facial Recovery. Middle: A patient with Ramsay Hunt syndrome demonstrates a pucker. Photograph courtesy of Michael J. Reilly, MD. Right: The right eye of a patient with zoster sine herpete cannot close due to lagophthalmos. Photograph courtesy of The Center for Facial Recovery.

We have included three examples of standardized grading scales at the end of this chapter. In addition to these formal assessments, functional activities such as inflating a balloon, blowing out a candle, or trying to whistle can also aid in assessing your current level of return.

Look to the Eye

The discomfort you experience when your eye can't close or blink is an important reason to see a facial palsy therapist.

As previously discussed, the facial nerve is responsible for eye closure. When the nerve is not able to send its usual signals to this sphincter muscle around the eye, called the orbicularis oculi, several complications can result. Most noticeable is a potentially serious condition called **lagophthalmos**, an inability of the affected eyelid to fully close.

There is research that indicates full eye closure is a good gauge of how long recovery will take and even how much recovery will occur. We've also found a correlation between the time until eye closure returns and the development of a tenacious complication called synkinesis.

If the lids of your affected eye cannot completely "kiss" or close, a facial palsy therapist can not only teach you proper self-care to prevent injury to the eye but can also help you work toward restoration of the muscle activity needed for normal eyelid function. (More on techniques to encourage eye closure is presented later in this chapter.)

In some cases, advanced interventions by an oculoplastic surgeon or a facial plastic surgeon might be warranted to assist eye closure (see Chapter 5.) A facial palsy therapist would be a good resource for selecting a specialist who could assess your specific needs. An interdisciplinary approach leads to the best outcomes.

Tackling Complications

Facial palsy therapy aims to improve the symmetrical appearance, function, and comfort of your entire face—both while talking or expressing emotion, and while your face is at rest. You and your therapist should discuss your rehabilitation goals and a rough timetable for seeing results.

Rehabilitation involves some crucial anatomical features besides the facial muscles and nerves that you'll need to know about as you begin the work of recovery. They include:

Fascia: *a sheath or flat bands of connective tissue located just below the skin.* Fascia can attach to, cover, or enclose muscle and organs. It's found throughout the body, including the face. If you've ever seen the thin, white membrane threaded between the skin and the breast of raw chicken, you know what fascia looks like.

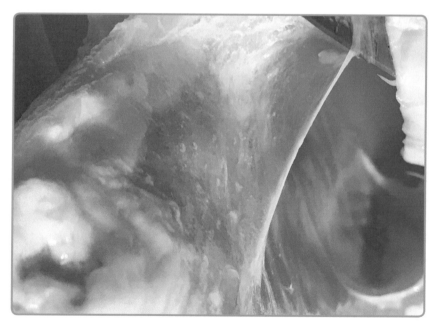

White patches and strands of fascia in a chicken breast. Photograph courtesy of Jodi Barth.

Fibrosis: *a thickening and scarring of connective tissues that can occur after an injury.* Lack of activity will cement the once-supple fibers into place. Special interventions can be helpful in freeing up this tissue.

Synkinesis: *a miswiring of regenerating facial nerves resulting in muscle movement that was not intended.* The connection between the nerves and muscles is a chemical one. The nerve delivers a chemical, called a neurotransmitter, that the muscle needs to activate. This process is like the connection between the internet and your computer. If the internet is out, your computer can't browse the web.

After facial palsy onset, activity in each branch of the facial nerve returns at a different rate. This means that each muscle region in need of that input receives it at a different rate, too.

Of all the activity that happens in the face, the brain prioritizes eye closure because it is a protective mechanism. Therefore, the eye area is shouting the loudest for the chemical to be delivered. If the nerves that are supposed to supply this power source are not yet functioning, any other nerve that has recovered faster will attempt to do so. This can lead to the abnormal nerve regeneration otherwise known as synkinesis.

When a person with synkinesis eats, their affected eye may blink with each chew. When they close their eye or frown, the corner of their mouth may pull up. And it can be a virtual symphony of synkinesis when they speak: the combination of their mouth pulling to one side while their eye winks and their cheek pulls can make the person feel as though their face has a mind of its own. Synkinesis can also cause neck and cheek tightness, watery eyes, chin dimpling, and the appearance of the affected eye being smaller than the other.

Synkinesis frequently develops in facial palsy patients who do not spontaneously recover in the first few weeks or months.

It is one of the hardest obstacles to overcome and does not improve on its own.

Electrical stimulation is often recommended for facial recovery. However, studies have found that this intervention may in fact interfere with neural regeneration, reinforce abnormal movement patterns (synkinesis), and impede progress.

People with facial palsy may also engage in overzealous, repetitive facial activity or aggressive massage trying to "revive" their weakened or paralyzed muscles. These harmful activities, which include chewing gum, should be avoided.

Facial palsy exercises should always be gentle, slow, and controlled! **See our at-home exercise regimen starting on page 67.**

Maximizing Results

Facial palsy therapy works best when multiple treatments are used to address the problem from different angles.

On a macro level, this involves a multidisciplinary team. A successful team approach may require the expertise of a facial plastic surgeon; oculoplastic surgeon; ENT (ear, nose, and throat specialist); neurologist; and physical, occupational, or speech therapist. Each member of this team should have specific training and experience in facial palsy treatment.

On a micro level, facial palsy responds best when a variety of modalities is employed, both traditional and unique. **The modalities presented here that we are categorizing as unique are not mainstream facial palsy treatment**. They are, however, based on established therapeutic procedures for use elsewhere on the body and have produced excellent clinical results for our facial rehabilitation patients.

If you can't find team-based physical therapy in your area, look for a provider who is excited by the idea of collaborating with other specialists. Similarly, if your therapist is open-minded, you might encourage them to explore these out-of-the-box adjunct treatments and evaluate how they affect recovery rates and patient satisfaction when used in conjunction with standard therapies.

Unique Interventions

Diagnostic Ultrasound Technology

Having an ultrasound assessment by an experienced facial palsy therapist is an innovative use of this established technology for treating facial paralysis. The standard technologies for evaluation of the facial nerve and the associated muscles are:

- dual-channel surface electromyography (EMG)
- surface electromyography (sEMG)
- nerve conduction velocity test (NCV)

Unlike these electro-diagnostic tests, ultrasound is noninvasive, not painful, cost-effective, and can be performed at acute onset and repeated on a regular basis to assess recovery.

Ultrasound allows the clinician and the patient to see any muscle contractions that aren't visible on the surface. For example, if there's no sign of your smile but a contraction shows up on the ultrasound screen when you try, you can celebrate that there is muscle activity. Similarly, ultrasound can show muscles misfiring, which could be an indication that synkinesis is developing. This allows the therapist to start interventions before aberrant muscle movement takes over.

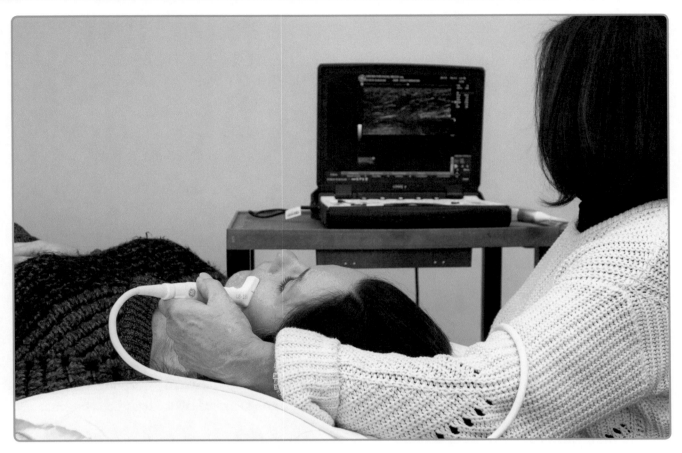

Ultrasound assessment. Photograph courtesy of The Center for Facial Recovery.

The Mirror Book™ and Face2Face Facial Palsy App

Many patients find it distressing and discouraging when performing mirror exercises. The Mirror Book addresses this problem. It is a groundbreaking rehabilitation device for neuromuscular reeducation. It provides real-time, twice-reflected visual feedback of the unaffected side of a person's face. In other words, when the patient looks in the mirror, it tricks the brain into seeing an approximation of their normal face. They experience less stress and are more encouraged as they perform their exercises than they would if they were watching their affected features move abnormally.

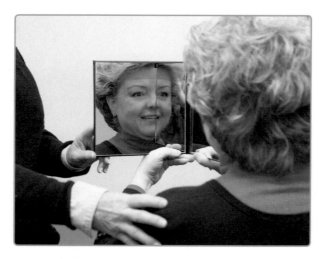

A patient performs Mirror Book therapy. Photograph courtesy of The Center for Facial Recovery.

Synkineedling®

The goal for treatment of synkinesis is to stop or decrease unwanted movements that occur with intentional and spontaneous movements. Your eye closing or squinting when you smile is an example. Synkineedling, pioneered by Jodi Barth, PT, is a synkinesis-targeting facial adaptation of a standard modality called dry needling. Dry needling can be used on the whole body as a treatment to restore proper function to locked, abnormally behaving muscles.

Synkineedling came into being after extensive ultrasound diagnostics on facial palsy patients revealed a pattern: muscles affected by synkinesis were usually surrounded by fibrotic tissue. Adapting dry needling to release this fibrosis has proven to be highly successful. (Patients may even *hear* that success: a popping or snapping sound is sometimes produced when the hardened tissue is released.)

Synkineedling interventions reduce the severity of synkinetic activity by at least 25 percent.

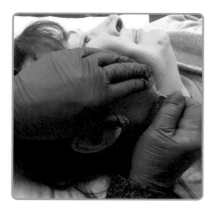

Synkineedling with a filament needle. Photograph courtesy of The Center for Facial Recovery.

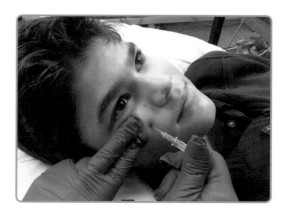

Synkineedling with a subcutaneous needle. Photograph courtesy of The Center for Facial Recovery.

IBBS™

IBBS is a technique that targets synkinesis. It is based on a procedure that debrides (breaks up) fibrosis in patients with carpal tunnel injuries. IBBS, which should be performed by a medical professional with extensive knowledge of facial anatomy, relies on high-definition ultrasound imaging to map out muscles that are being restricted by fibrosis; the fibrotic tissue is then broken up, leaving muscle tissue free to expand. Patients often see improved movement within hours to days. Facial palsy therapy must be initiated immediately following the procedure and continued on a regular basis. This includes neuromuscular reeducation and manual manipulation, which will optimize the effects of the release.

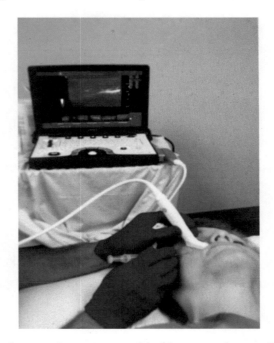

A patient with synkinesis due to intractable fibrosis undergoes IBBS. Because the needle is inserted deeper into the tissue than in synkineedling, a numbing agent is administered first. The face may bruise but recovery is otherwise immediate.

Vasopneumatic Therapy

This modality, also called a negative pressure device, uses a principle similar to cupping.

The device momentarily pulls or "sucks up" the surface skin along with intermediate and deep layers. Pressure is then released, the treated area recedes, and the wand is moved to the next target area. It all happens quickly and rhythmically and is largely pain-free. The treatment helps relieve muscle spasms, release restricted tissue, and increase circulation.

Patients can purchase a commercially available skincare device that works in a similar manner. It can be used to improve circulation at home in between therapy sessions with the professional unit.

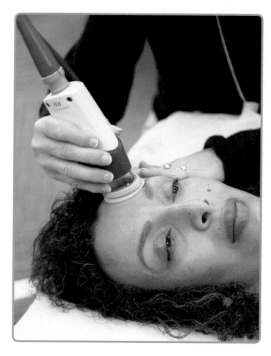

The suction sensation during vasopneumatic therapy is generally painless.
Photograph courtesy of The Center for Facial Recovery.

Radial Pulse Therapy

Radial pulse therapy for the face was inspired by its traditional use on patients with plantar fasciitis. It is a painless, noninvasive technique that provides high-energy pulses that promote myofascial release and improved tissue quality.

With both vasopneumatic pump and radial pulse therapies, tissue can be manipulated at a deeper level than with manual techniques. Patients can immediately feel a difference in the amount of muscle movement and decreased tissue thickness in the treated area.

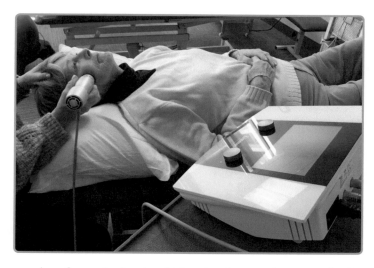

Patients frequently refer to the loud radial pulse therapy device as the "jackhammer."
Photograph courtesy of The Center for Facial Recovery.

Light Therapy

Exposure to this treatment's infrared light helps cells regenerate or repair themselves and improves the circulation of oxygen-rich blood. Light therapy helps deep tissue in treated areas heal faster and promotes pain relief.

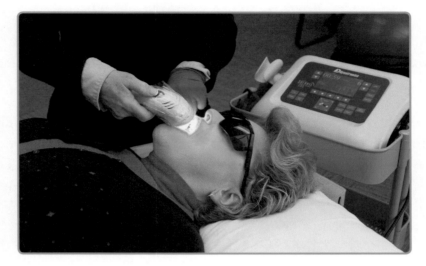

Light therapy in progress. Photograph courtesy of The Center for Facial Recovery.

Laser Therapy

Laser therapy accelerates the body's own natural healing process through photobiostimulation. With this modality, red and near-infrared light is passed over affected areas to "excite" cells. This increases circulation and reduces pain and inflammation.

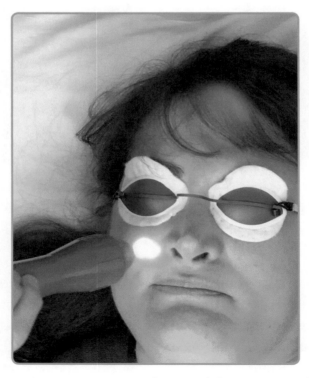

Laser therapy in progress. Photograph by Luis Miranda.

Kinesiology Taping Techniques

Kinesiology taping techniques involve placing a thin, stretchy therapeutic tape onto the skin to manipulate muscles and help retrain the brain to learn normal muscle function. This treatment has long been used by physical therapists, but it is not widely applied in facial palsy therapy.

This technique can be used to provide sensory input to the face, which promotes movement. It can stimulate a muscle or decrease its activity, increase circulation, decrease swelling, diminish scarring, and more. It is a natural adjunct to manual therapy and neuromuscular reeducation.

One example of kinesiology taping's use in facial palsy: A patient whose eye can't fully close can place a strip of tape under the lower eyelid and gently anchor it to the outside corner of the eye area. This provides support to allow the two lids to "kiss," which is necessary for effective eye closure. The same technique can also pull a weak lower lip muscle up and out to improve an asymmetrical smile and improve speech. Your therapist can show you how to correctly apply the tape.

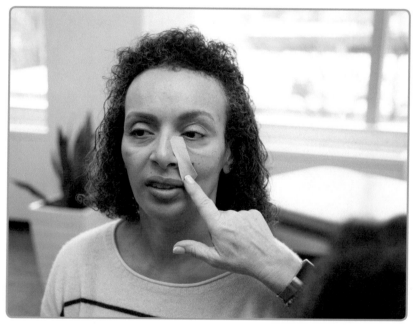

A patient has kinesiology tape applied to promote upper lip activity. Photograph courtesy of The Center for Facial Recovery.

Telehealth Sessions

The same technology that now allows doctors to diagnose the flu in a patient a hundred miles away can bring the specialized care of a facial palsy therapist to anyone with a computer and internet connection. Specialized software programs that protect your health information allow the therapist to evaluate, coach, and instruct you in real time. While hands-on adjunct treatments can only be done in the office, the technology allows for a full evaluation and facial grading on a standardized grading scale. It can also provide video recording of facial movement and appearance for progress monitoring, tailored instruction in facial exercises, and even coordination with your other healthcare providers.

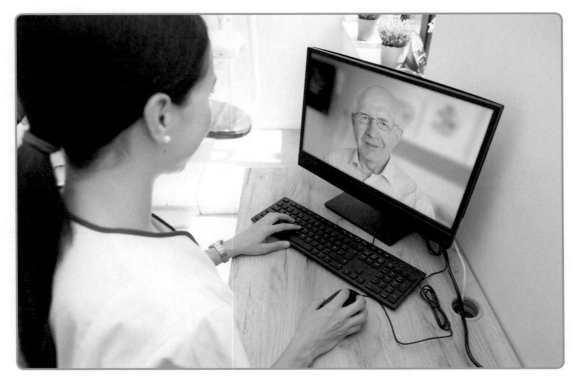

Facial palsy treatment conducted through telehealth sessions can be highly effective. Photograph by Proxima Studios / Shutterstock.

STANDARD INTERVENTIONS

Soft Tissue Massage

This modality promotes tissue regeneration and reduces scar tissue and swelling; pumps oxygen and nutrients into tissues and vital organs, improving circulation; reduces spasms and cramping; relaxes and softens injured and overused muscles; and releases endorphins to reduce pain.

Neuromuscular Reeducation

This technique consists of slow, deliberate exercises to improve brain neuroplasticity. Neuromuscular reeducation is a crucial part of overcoming synkinesis. For facial palsy patients, this can include EMG biofeedback, mirror therapy, mime, and ultrasound-guided exercises.

Cranio-sacral Therapy

Cranio-sacral therapy is another technique to improve blood flow to the affected area, which in turn decreases inflammation and improves mobility. The traditional approach to this therapy centers around fascial release of the cranium. Because this fascia is connected to fascia on the face, tightness in the cranial region could limit muscle activity, range of motion, and blood flow on the face below. When adapted for facial palsy patients, the emphasis is on using massage to gently unwind and release fascial strain under the scalp.

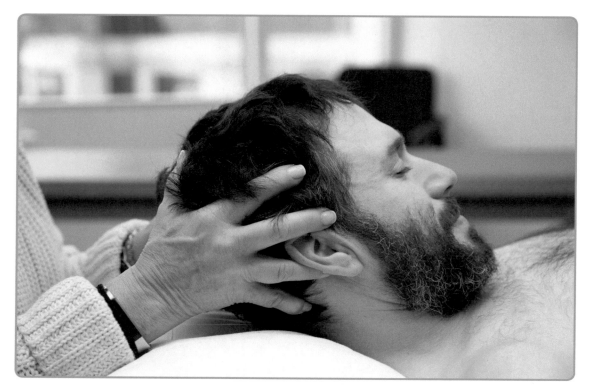

A patient receives relaxing cranio-facial therapy following adjunct treatments and facial exercises. Photograph courtesy of The Center for Facial Recovery.

Biofeedback

Neuromuscular facial retraining using EMG feedback is effective in improving facial movement and minimizing synkinesis. It provides immediate feedback to the patient. See Chapter 8 for more information.

Neurotoxins

Facial palsy patients often benefit from seeing a physician who specializes in the treatment of facial palsy with the use of neurotoxins. (Botox®, Dysport®, and Xeomin® are brand-name neurotoxins.) When done in team-based coordination with physical therapy, the therapist can teach the patient how to reeducate the muscles in a more normal environment, one that isn't waylaid by unnatural tightness or aberrant movement. For example, a neurotoxin injection in the neck's platysma helps release its pull on the lower lip.

Facial Exercises and At-Home Therapy

The following exercise regimen is offered as a preview of what facial palsy treatments may consist of and should be carried out only when under the care of a qualified physical therapist or other healthcare professional with experience treating facial palsy.

Your therapist will show you which exercises are appropriate for the stage of facial palsy you are in. There are three stages:

Flaccid Paralysis

- *Condition*: no tone or movement in facial muscles, no ability to generate expressions of emotions, poor facial symmetry, difficulty with eye closure, and difficulty with eating and drinking.
- *Treatment priority*: self-care education, eye care, gentle massage, and targeted stretching for the opposite side.

Paresis

- *Condition*: increase in tone, starting to see muscle movement, somewhat improved symmetry, and no synkinesis.
- *Treatment priority*: neuromuscular reeducation, slow and controlled activity with minimized overactivity of the unaffected side, continued gentle massage, and targeted stretching.

Synkinesis

- *Condition*: significantly increased muscle tone and abnormal muscle patterns.
- *Treatment priority*: stretching, massage, neuromuscular reeducation, slow and controlled activity with minimized overactivity of the unaffected side, and manual therapy focused on improving tissue quality.

PT Points to Remember

When performing any facial palsy exercise, follow these guidelines:

- ✓ Exercises should be slow and controlled. Slow and steady wins the race!

- ✓ Facial palsy exercises are a marathon, not a sprint. Be patient.

- ✓ Prioritize quality over quantity.

- ✓ Never exercise to the point of fatigue.

- ✓ Exercises should not hurt or make you feel uncomfortable afterward.

- ✓ Don't get discouraged if you feel motion but don't see it. Feeling muscle activity is the first stage of the recovery process.

Tips and Tricks

Prep facial muscles with a warm compress before stretching, massaging, or exercising for maximum benefit. Massage should precede exercises.

S-t-r-e-t-c-h! All facial palsy patients, regardless of where they are in their recovery, can benefit from simple, regular, focused stretching of the face and/or neck muscles to address tightness and prevent or minimize fibrosis. All stretches should be performed slowly and gently—never to the point of pain—and repeated as often throughout the day as is practical. Note: Never pull down on your lower eyelid!

This is your time to help your healing process. Try to perform your exercises in a quiet, relaxed environment free from family distractions.

Perform relaxation breathing before and during exercises to help reduce the anxiety that may be generated by looking at or thinking about your face. Sit comfortably with your back straight; breathe in deeply through your nose; exhale through your mouth, pushing out as much air as you can while contracting your abdominal muscles. Continue for five minutes.

Consider trying one of the multiple apps available to guide you through relaxation and mindfulness exercises that can help with minimizing stress and reducing synkinetic activity.

Weave exercises into your daily routine—after brushing your teeth, while watching television, or while carpooling if you are not the driver, for example. Set your smartphone alarm to remind you.

Sleep wearing a nasal strip on your nose to separate your nasal passages, which may have been impaired by your facial palsy.

Look to your facial palsy side with your eyes if you feel eye synkinesis when performing exercises. (In other words, if you have left-side facial palsy, look left. For right-side facial palsy, look right.)

Make the Most of Massage

Massage feels great and is great for you. Here are suggestions for making the most of this important healing treatment.

Understand the purpose. The goal of massage is to make muscles more pliable for exercises, improve circulation, and prevent interstitial fluids from pooling and hardening into fibrosis.

Massage both sides of the face in small, circular motions using the pads of your fingers. Your therapist can guide you in specific massage techniques unique to your condition.

Add warmth to the mix whenever possible. Ideal times to massage are while showering or taking a bath. Applying a warm compress also helps.

Commercial massage creams are a nice aid because they stay silky and are not absorbed as quickly as regular creams or lotions, but they are not a requirement.

Massaging your face and scalp several times a day is very beneficial, but your regimen must work with your schedule.

When you massage your face or have someone else do it, we recommend these directions:

1. From the hairline down to the eye
2. From the cheekbone up to the eye
3. From the ear toward the nose
4. From the chin up toward the corner of the mouth and toward the nose

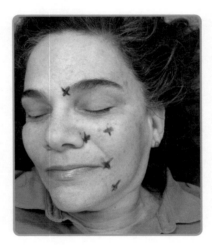

Areas marked with an X indicate where facial palsy patients tend to have the most tightness, thickness, and pain. Massaging and stretching here will improve tissue quality. Photograph courtesy of The Center for Facial Recovery.

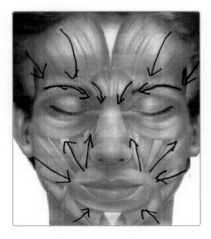

Massage in the direction of the arrows. Massage both sides so you are aware of the difference in tissue texture between your involved side and your uninvolved side. This will tell you where you need to concentrate your efforts. Illustration courtesy of The Center for Facial Recovery.

Now your muscles are looser and optimally primed for exercises!

Help Your Eye Learn to Close Again

Bathe your eye area with warm soaks for 5 to 10 minutes, 2 to 3 times a day.

Massages

1. Gently massage downward on your forehead toward your eyebrows as you close your eyes. Continue for two minutes.
2. Massage above the inner corner of the eyebrow in a downward motion, utilizing firm pressure to release the thickness of tissue under your fingers. Continue for two minutes.

Stretches

Remember: Never stretch your lower lid downward.

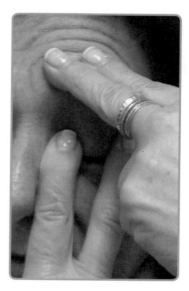

Stretch #1 to promote eye closure. Photograph by Maria Mihalik.

1. With eyes closed, gently place one finger on either side of your top eyelid, avoiding the eyeball, while you stretch the eyebrow region up with the other hand. Hold for 30 seconds, repeat 3 times.
2. Place two fingers along your hairline and stretch up while using another two fingers just below them to pull down. Start at the midline and work toward your ear. Perform this slowly 5 times.
3. Pull down the top of your ear as you push up on the scalp area above. Hold for 30 seconds, repeat 3 times.
4. Pull your ear forward with one hand while you stabilize your scalp behind the ear with the other hand. Hold for 30 seconds, repeat 3 times.

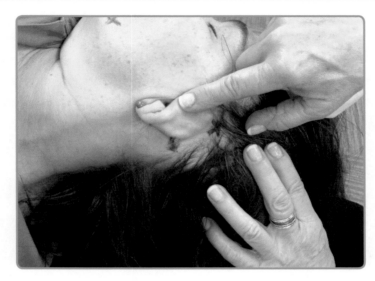

Stretch #4 for eye closure. Photograph courtesy of The Center for Facial Recovery.

Neuromuscular Reeducation

1. While sitting up straight, look down with your eyes without moving your head. Close your eyes, hold for 5 seconds, repeat 10 times.
2. Assist eye closure by gently pushing down at your eyebrow as you close your eye.
3. Gently push upward just below your lower eyelid as you close your eyes. Hold for 5 seconds, repeat 10 times.

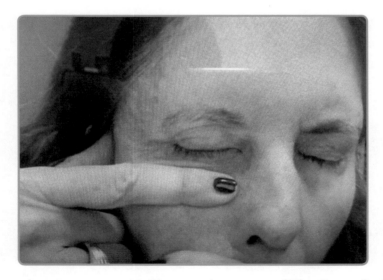

Neuromuscular reeducation exercise #3. Photograph courtesy of The Center for Facial Recovery.

Control Eye Synkinesis

Massage

Using a slow, circular motion, gently massage your temple area on your affected side as you perform facial expressions or while eating or drinking.

Neuromuscular Reeducation

1. If you feel your eye closing when performing facial expression exercises, gently close both eyes, hold for 5 seconds, and then continue the activity as you gently open your eyes.
2. When performing facial exercises, stop just before you feel the synkinesis kicking in, even if you are only able to accomplish a very small motion.

Decrease Eye Tearing While Eating

1. Eat slowly, take smaller bites, and drink lots of fluids with your meal.
2. Slowly massage your jaw area in a clockwise direction for one to two minutes.

Improve Your Smile

Stretches

1. Stretch your platysma, the muscle running from below your collar bone to the mid-part of the face. Pull down on the skin at your collar bone on your affected side, turn your head toward the opposite side, and protrude your jaw. Hold for 30 seconds, repeat 3 times. If this causes discomfort, don't protrude the jaw.
2. Hook your thumb under your affected top lip as you stretch the lip downward from the outside with your index finger. Hold for 30 seconds, repeat 3 times.
3. Place your right thumb in your affected cheek while your index finger rests on the outside of your cheek. Stretch the corner of your mouth gently toward your unaffected ear. Hold for 30 seconds, repeat 3 times.
4. Place a soft ping-pong ball in your cheek to stretch out the area of tightness, which could be on the involved or uninvolved side.
5. Use a soft-coated baby spoon to stretch the inside of your lip, top and bottom.

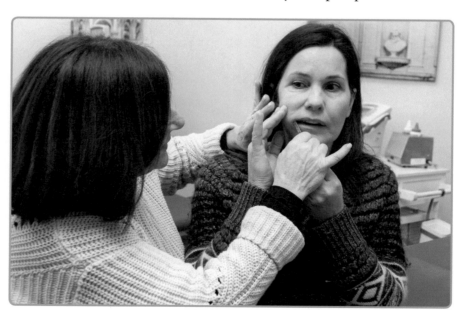

A baby spoon is helpful for stretching the inside of the mouth.
Photograph courtesy of The Center for Facial Recovery.

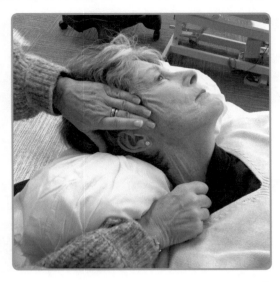

Stretching the platysma. Photograph courtesy of the Center for Facial Recovery.

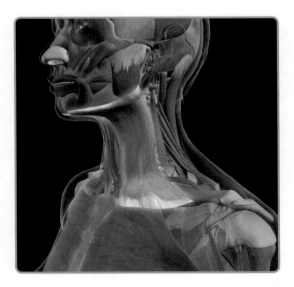

The platysma muscle (in bright orange). Image by Hank Grebe / Shutterstock.

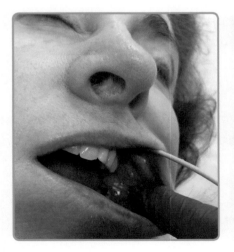 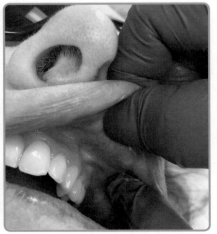

After one session of stretching the mouth and cheek area, a patient shows remarkable increase in tissue mobility. Photograph courtesy of The Center for Facial Recovery.

Neuromuscular Reeducation

1. Place your hands on both cheeks and feel how the tissue moves when you go into a smile. Assist your involved side so it feels like it is moving like your uninvolved side. Hold for 5 seconds, repeat 10 times.
2. Go into a closed-mouth smile while resisting movement in the unaffected corner of your mouth. Hold for 5 seconds, repeat 10 times.
3. Go into a gentle, open-mouth smile while resisting movement on the unaffected side of your mouth. Hold for 5 seconds, repeat 10 times.
4. Place two fingers at either corner of your mouth and gently assist your pucker. Assist your involved side so it feels like it is moving like your uninvolved side. Hold for 5 seconds, repeat 10 times.
5. Place two fingers above your top lip under your nose and gently assist your snarl upward. Assist your involved side so it feels like it is moving like your uninvolved side. Hold for 5 seconds, repeat 10 times.
6. Slowly and without engaging your affected eye, go into a small, closed-lip "Mona Lisa" smile. Hold for 5 seconds, repeat 10 times.
7. Whistle happy birthday, even if you were never able to whistle. If you feel your affected eye tighten up, gently close both eyes to assist in releasing the tightness there.
8. Gently puff air behind your lips. Hold for 5 seconds, repeat 10 times.
9. Using your soft ping-pong ball in the unaffected cheek, try reading out loud to reduce the motion of the unaffected side and optimize activity of the affected side.

Decrease a Pronounced Nasolabial Fold (the curved line on your cheek running from your nose to your mouth)

Massage

Massage the pronounced fold from side to side (toward and then away from your nose) until it feels less tender and has more mobility.

Stretch

Place your finger inside your top lip by your canine tooth and stretch the under part of the lip outward away from the teeth. Hold for 5 seconds, repeat 10 times.

Neuromuscular Reeducation

Place a strip of kinesiology tape over the fold, starting at the top and anchoring it where the fold ends by your lip. Try to wear it for a few hours a day, provided it is tolerable and doesn't irritate your skin. (See photo on page 64.)

Strengthen Your Jaw Muscles

1. Place your tongue on the roof of your mouth; gently open your mouth without the tongue losing contact. Hold for 5 seconds, repeat 10 times.
2. Click your tongue 10 times.

3. With the tip of your tongue on the roof of your mouth, draw 5 circles clockwise and 5 counterclockwise.

Diminish Dimples in Your Chin

Massage

Massage your chin side to side for 2 minutes.

Neuromuscular Reeducation

1. Pinch the sides of your chin with your thumb and index finger; squeeze and go into a pout. Hold for 5 seconds, repeat 10 times.
2. Roll your lower lip in. Hold for 5 seconds, repeat 10 times.

Improve Your Posture to Benefit Your Face

Perform these subtle moves when commuting on the subway, standing in line at the store or bank, etc.

1. Squeeze your buttocks. Hold for 5 seconds, repeat 10 times.
2. Squeeze your shoulder blades back. Hold for 5 seconds, repeat 10 times.
3. Pull your belly button toward your spine. Hold for 5 seconds, repeat 10 times.

———————

Always hold your cellphone, tablet, or print book up to face level—don't look down!
Looking down is an insidious cause of neck pain, which can affect facial muscles.

———————

End Your Day on a Good Note for Your Face

1. Repeat relaxation breathing. Sit comfortably with your back straight. Breathe in deeply through your nose. Exhale through your mouth, pushing out as much air as you can while contracting your abdominal muscles. Continue for 5 minutes.
2. Soothe your eyes and face with a warm compress.
3. Close your eyes. Gently massage your face and scalp as instructed previously for 5 minutes.

Gallery

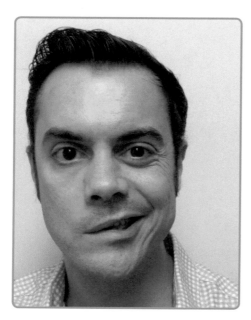

Patient A, presenting with Ramsay Hunt syndrome.

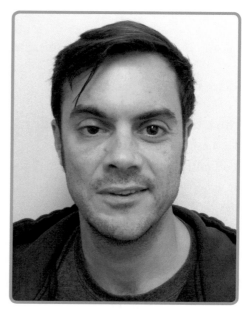

Patient A after 19 months of treatment.

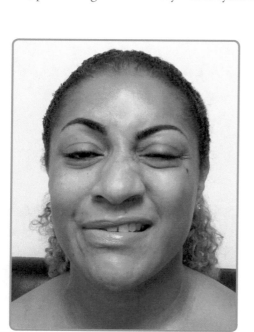

Patient B, a patient with Bell's palsy.

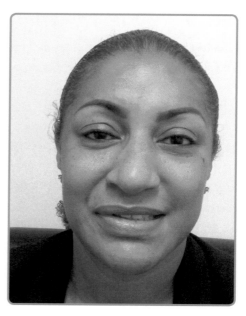

Patient B after 2 years of treatment.

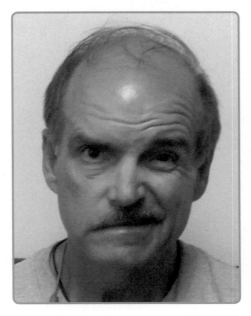

Patient C, presenting with Bell's palsy.

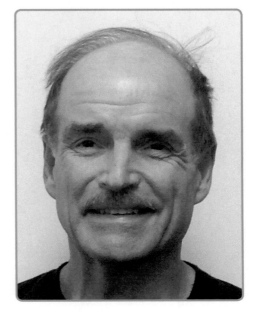

Patient C after 8 months of treatment.

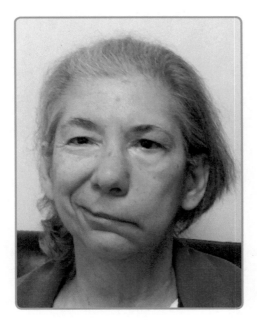

Patient D, a patient with zoster sine herpete.

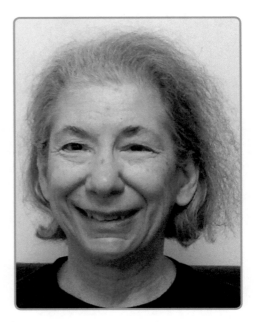

Patient D after 16 months of treatment.

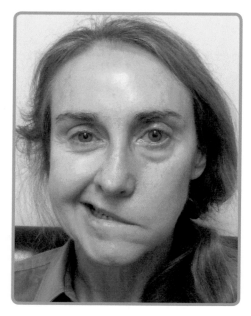

Patient E, presenting with surgical injury to facial nerve.

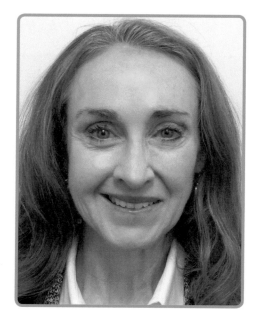

Patient E after 18 months of treatment.

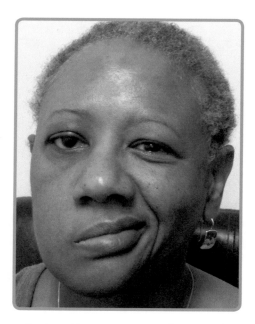

Patient F, presenting with surgical injury to facial nerve.

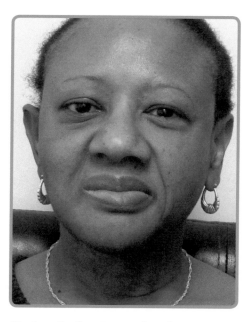

Patient F after 9 months of treatment.

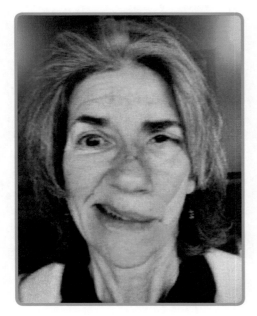

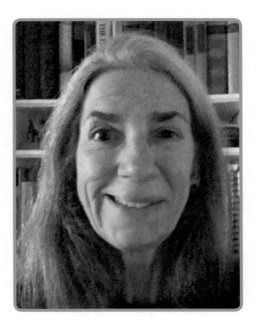

Patient G, presenting with facial palsy after accidental injury to facial nerve. Photograph courtesy of the patient.

Patient G after 5½ years of treatment. Photograph courtesy of the patient.

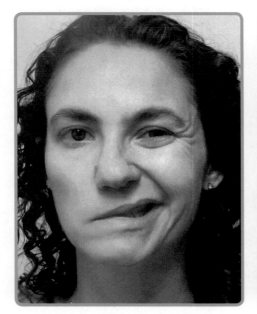

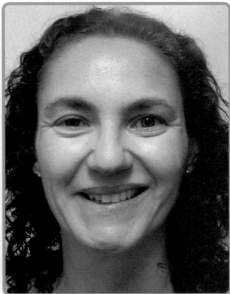

Patient H, before and after 15 months of treatment for Ramsay Hunt syndrome.

Sunnybrook Facial Grading System

Resting Symmetry

Compared to normal side

Eye (choose one only)
- normal ☐ 0
- narrow ☐ 1
- wide ☐ 1
- eyelid surgery ☐ 1

Cheek (naso-labial fold)
- normal ☐ 0
- absent ☐ 2
- less pronounced ☐ 1
- more pronounced ☐ 1

Mouth
- normal ☐ 0
- corner drooped ☐ 1
- corner pulled up/out ☐ 1

Total **0**

Resting Symmetry score

Total X 5 **0**

Patient's Name _____

Diagnosis _____

1/20/2020
Date _____

Symmetry of Voluntary Movement

Degree of muscle EXCURSION compared to normal side

Standard Expressions	Unable to initiate movement	Initiates slight movement	Initiates movement with mild excursion	Movement almost complete	Movement complete	
Brow lift (FRO)	☐ 1	☐ 2	☐ 3	☐ 4	☐ 5	**0**
Geltle eye closure (OCS)	☐ 1	☐ 2	☐ 3	☐ 4	☐ 5	**0**
Open mouth Smile (SYG/RIS)	☐ 1	☐ 2	☐ 3	☐ 4	☐ 5	**0**
Snarl (LLA/LLS)	☐ 1	☐ 2	☐ 3	☐ 4	☐ 5	**0**
Lip Pucker (OOS/OOI)	☐ 1	☐ 2	☐ 3	☐ 4	☐ 5	**0**
	Gross Asymmetry	Severe Asymmetry	Moderate Asymmetry	Mild Asymmetry	Normal Asymmetry	Total **0**

Voluntary movement score: Total X 4 **0**

Synkinesis

Rate the degree of INVOLUNTARY MUSCLE CONTRACTION assocaited with each expression

	NONE: no synkinesis or mass movement	MILD: slight synkinesis of one or more muscles	MODERATE: obvious synkinesis of one or more muscles	SEVERE: disfiguring synkinesis/ gross mass movement of several muscles	
Brow lift (FRO)	☐ 0	☐ 1	☐ 2	☐ 3	**0**
Geltle eye closure (OCS)	☐ 0	☐ 1	☐ 2	☐ 3	**0**
Open mouth Smile (SYG/RIS)	☐ 0	☐ 1	☐ 2	☐ 3	**0**
Snarl (LLA/LLS)	☐ 0	☐ 1	☐ 2	☐ 3	**0**
Lip Pucker (OOS/OOI)	☐ 0	☐ 1	☐ 2	☐ 3	**0**

Synkinesis score: Total **0**

Vol mov't score **0** − Resting symm score **0** − Synk score **0** = Composite Score: **0**

© 1992 Ross BG, Fradet G, Nedzelski JM
Sunnybrook Health Science Centre
Permission not required to produce unaltered

House-Brackmann facial nerve grading system

Grade I - Normal
Normal facial function in all areas

Grade II - Slight Dysfunction
Gross: slight weakness noticeable on close inspection; may have very slight synkinesis
At rest: normal symmetry and tone
Motion: forehead - moderate to good function; eye - complete closure with minimum effort; mouth - slight asymmetry.

Grade III - Moderate Dysfunction
Gross: obvious but not disfiguring difference between two sides; noticeable but not severe synkinesis, contracture, and/or hemi-facial spasm.
At rest: normal symmetry and tone
Motion: forehead - slight to moderate movement; eye - complete closure with effort; mouth - slightly weak with maximum effort.

Grade IV - Moderate Severe Dysfunction
Gross: obvious weakness and/or disfiguring asymmetry
At rest: normal symmetry and tone
Motion: forehead - none; eye - incomplete closure; mouth - asymmetric with maximum effort.

Grade V - Severe Dysfunction
Gross: only barely perceptible motion
At rest: asymmetry
Motion: forehead - none; eye - incomplete closure; mouth - slight movement

Grade VI - Total Paralysis
No movement

House, J.W., Brackmann, D.E. Facial nerve grading system. Otolaryngol. Head Neck Surg, [93] 146–147. 1985.

FACE Instrument
date:

The following statements are about how you think your face is moving.
You may have answered these or similar questions before.

Please answer all questions as best you can.
If you have problems on both sides, respond regarding your more affected side.

	Question	Score
1	When I try to move my face, I have difficulty on:	

note: 1= one side, 2 = 2 sides, 0= I have no difficulty

For questions 2-4, use the following rating scale to complete the sentence:

1 = not at all
2 = only if I concentrate
3 = a little
4 = almost normally
5 = normally

	Question	Score
2	When I smile, the corner of my mouth goes up	
3	I can raise my eyebrow	
4	When I pucker my lips, the affected side of my mouth moves	

For questions 5-13, use the following rating scale to complete the sentence:

1 = all of the time
2 = most of the time
3 = some of the time
4 = a little of the time
5 = none of the time

	Question	Score
5	Parts of my face feel tight, worn out, or uncomfortable	
6	My affected eye feels dry, irritated, or scratchy	
7	When I move my face, I feel tension, pain, or spasm	
8	I use eye drops or ointment in my affected eye	
9	My affected eye is wet or has tears in it	
10	I act differently around other people because of my face	
11	People treat me differently because of my face	
12	I have problems moving food around in my mouth	
13	I have problems with drooling, or keeping food/drink in my mouth	

All photographs in gallery courtesy of The Center for Facial Recovery except where noted.

CHAPTER 8
Biofeedback: Mind Over Matter

Emily Perlman, LCPC, BCB, SMC-C

"You can feel movement better when you can see it." —Emma

Biofeedback is a noninvasive, drug-free treatment modality that teaches people how to use their mind to gain control over physiological processes in their bodies that are typically involuntary. Involuntary processes mean they normally happen without having to think about them. Breathing, feeling pain or anxiety, blinking, and sweating are examples.

You'll find the procedure itself to be painless and simple. It doesn't require any preparation on your part. You'll simply be connected by electrodes and wires (called leads) to one of several different types of biofeedback equipment that measures and feeds back physiological information to you and the person monitoring the session.

Biofeedback technologies include:

- electroencephalograph (EEG) to monitor brain waves
- electrocardiograph (ECG) to measure heart rate
- electrodermograph (EDG) to measure the sweat response
- surface electromyograph (sEMG) to read the electrical activity of muscle contraction.

During the procedure, a certified biofeedback therapist will show you a monitor that displays lines, bars, gamelike graphics, or audio feedback in response to what is happening on the skin and under the skin. By watching the screen, you'll become aware of the automatic muscle response and learn to change it in a way that improves function. You may do this by visualizing the correct muscle activity and then attempting to create the same movement. In this way, you activate the brain to send a clear signal to the area you are working on and subtly change what is happening.

The Ultrasound Alternative

While sEMG has been the go-to test for monitoring muscle contraction, **ultrasound imaging is proving to be as effective and, for many people, even more motivating.** Rather than using lines or lights to graphically represent muscle activity, ultrasound's black-and-white imaging shows the muscles themselves as they contract (or fail to, as with paralysis). You can see on the screen the difference between the affected side and the non-affected side so you can try to make the affected side simulate what the good side has done. Both technologies, however, allow you to see the actual effect your effort is having on your face.

Smaller Is Harder

People with facial weakness or synkinesis can use these tools to perform an exercise they are having trouble with (lifting the eyebrow without pulling the lower face, for instance) and watch how the muscles' movements are reflected on the monitor. This allows for powering up, toning down, or otherwise redirecting the activity of the muscle that is involuntarily contributing to the abnormal movement or appearance of the face.

The effort is not easy: isolating such small muscles is much harder than targeting one in the shoulder or leg. Marathon runners have commented that facial exercises are more difficult then training for a marathon. But through this continued practice, patients are eventually able to create positive "muscle memory" that produces the desired result without concerted effort. In doing so, they measurably reduce synkinesis and ease facial tightness.

Facial Palsy Is Stressful

Stress is a common struggle for people with facial palsy. They wonder if they will ever get better and fear they will not. Studies show that biofeedback is an excellent tool to reduce pain, stress, and anxiety. These complications can lead to tightness in shoulder and neck muscles, which in turn can contribute to generalized tightness on the affected side of the face.

In addition to addressing muscle tension, the biofeedback instrument can monitor heart rate, skin conductance, and hand temperature, all of which are physiological readings of the stress response. Armed with this information, you can learn how to reduce heart rate, improve body temperature, and relax muscles. This interconnectedness adds another dimension to biofeedback's appropriateness for treating facial palsy.

It's important to note that if you begin biofeedback therapy, regardless of the reason, you will likely need to commit to an average of two to three months of sessions. And, most important for facial palsy patients, biofeedback should be used in conjunction with other treatment modalities— especially facial palsy physical therapy—for maximum effect.

Seeking Treatment

Biofeedback treatment is covered by some insurance companies. Its use in lowering blood pressure and as an alternative method of pain management is increasing the availability of plan coverage.

Since many biofeedback specialists are also trained in physical therapy, nursing, psychology, or other healthcare fields, the treatment is frequently offered at physical therapy clinics, hospitals, and medical centers.

Biofeedback-based apps, programs, and wearables that work through smartphones and computers are offered by a growing number of companies purporting to help relax muscles, improve breathing, lower heart rate and blood pressure, and diminish stress levels. Aside from trying reputably reviewed products to reduce tension, people with facial palsy should work with certified facial-anatomy technicians in a professional setting.

Consider the following ways to find a qualified biofeedback provider:

- Ask a neurologist or primary care doctor for a referral.
- Ask a physical therapist who treats facial palsy; if they do not perform the service, they will often know someone with relevant experience.
- Insurance plans that cover the treatment can also provide referrals to professionals in their network, but you will need to ask the provider directly about their familiarity with facial palsy.
- The Association for Applied Psychophysiology and Biofeedback (www.aapb.org), under the "Consumer Warning" tab, offers insights on licensing and guidance on biofeedback products. It also has a nationwide directory of providers.
- Biofeedback Certification International Alliance also has a nationwide directory of certified providers at www.bcia.org.

Biofeedback at Home

All you need for at-home biofeedback is a mirror and some small, round stickers. (We call them dots.)

Place a dot on an area that moves in an undesirable way. For example, adhere the dot under your affected eye and then pucker your lips or smile. Keep this movement slow and controlled to minimize any involuntary movement under your eye.

Hint: You can place a dot under your uninvolved area to see what normal motion there looks like during a pucker or smile. Then, slowly try again to recreate the motion on your affected side.

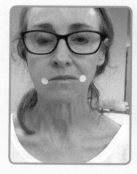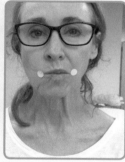

A patient uses stickers to help muscles on her affected side recreate the movement of her unaffected side. Photographs courtesy of The Center for Facial Recovery.

CHAPTER 9

New Frontiers for the Face: Regenerative Medicine and Hydrodissection

Nathan R. Yokel, MD, MPH, MBA

Medical researchers and physicians expanding the boundaries of traditional medicine are using creative approaches to heal cells, tissues, and organs in the body that are damaged due to illnesses or injuries. Several technologies that fall under the umbrella of regenerative or reparative medicine, as well as injection procedures called hydrodissection, show intriguing promise for someday joining the small arsenal of treatments for facial paralysis due to seventh cranial nerve trauma.

Regenerative Medicine

Regenerative medicine is based on the concept of injecting or implanting a substance into an injured area to stimulate an inflammatory or healing response. It has been used on both acute and chronic injuries throughout the body.

The following technologies are ripe for further exploration in the face.

Prolotherapy (or proliferative therapy). This treatment involves injecting an irritant solution of natural substances such as dextrose (a medical-grade sugar), saline, or glycerin into injured tissue. Hypertonic dextrose solutions, for one, act by dehydrating cells at the injection site. This leads to mild local tissue trauma that triggers the body's healing response: as cells called granulocytes and macrophages rush to repair and strengthen the affected region (Banks, 1991) (Hashemi, et al 2015), there is an increase in blood supply and growth factors, both of which are essential for repairing ligaments, tendons, and joints.

A subset of prolotherapy, called **neural prolotherapy**, uses perineural subcutaneous injections (injections just under the skin) of dextrose or other substances to improve nerve function and pain.

Neural prolotherapy works by reducing the tension from adjacent fascial or connective tissue compression that was causing nerve swelling and inhibited flow of nerve growth factors (Lyftogt 2007) (Weglein 2011) (Bennett, et al 1988). This helps in many ways, as the nerve that supplies a joint will often also supply the muscles that move the joint and the skin that covers it (Hilton 1879). With multiple rounds of neural prolotherapy, patients can achieve long-term calming of painful and dysfunctional nerves (Lyftogt 2007).

Prolotherapy can be an effective treatment for conditions affecting pain and functionality of the face. However, it is likely not potent enough to cause direct, significant change in nerve regrowth or recovery. Augmenting prolotherapy with mechanical hydrodissection (see page 87) merits consideration with nerve injury of the face.

Platelet-rich plasma (PRP) therapy. PRP consists of drawing blood from the patient, separating it into layers of plasma, platelets, and red blood cells, and then injecting just the platelets and associated growth and signaling factors back into the affected area. Chemical messengers in the platelets' alpha granules trigger cells to repair damage.

Clinical studies have shown that PRP patients can experience positive changes in pain and function. Studies have also shown that electromyography (EMG) parameters for muscle function in many peripheral nerve injuries and palsies were improved after ultrasound-guided injection of platelet-rich plasma into and right next to nerves throughout the body (Sánchez, et al 2018).

Some common nerve entrapments and injuries that have been studied include median neuropathy in the wrist or carpal tunnel syndrome causing hand pain and weakness (Wu, et al 2017) (Kuo, et al 2017); the radial nerve in the forearm causing wrist weakness (García de Cortázar, et al 2018); and the common peroneal nerve causing lower leg pain and foot drop (Sánchez, et al 2014). The use of platelet-rich plasma in epidural injections to treat lower back and neck nerve and radiating pain as well as injured and degenerative discs of the spine is becoming more common, with additional studies being published every year (Mohammed and Yu 2018).

PRP is also being used intraoperatively to bridge nerve gaps or wrap around injured nerves to allow better healing after they are moved to provide function to a new area (Kuffler 2014) (Hibner, et al 2012).

Regarding facial palsy, use of platelet-rich plasma to augment surgical repair of facial nerve injuries has been studied in animals (Farrag, et al 2007) (Cho, et al 2010), but more research is needed in human patients. (Most published work on humans has been limited to case studies and reports.) Platelet-rich plasma treatments have also been used to treat facial pain associated with trigeminal neuralgia (Doss 2012). Case studies have also noted use of PRP to aid in recovery from Bell's palsy (Seffer, et al 2017).

There is growing evidence and clinical success surrounding the use of platelet-rich plasma injections not just for many peripheral nerve injuries but also to improve nerves and musculoskeletal dysfunction in the face. So a foundation exists for continued investigation in patients with facial pain and palsy.

Bone marrow aspirate concentrate and microfragmented adipose (fat) grafts. A wide variety of injuries and conditions throughout the body can be treated with these procedures. (Autologous means the patient is both the donor and recipient.) The patient's own bone marrow or fat is harvested, cleaned, washed, reshaped, and in some cases concentrated to make material that, guided by ultrasound, is then injected (or used during surgery) to help heal or repair the affected area.

When placed in the injury site, the harvested material releases beneficial chemical messengers and growth factors. Healing may also be due to the replacement of motor neurons (nerves that affect movement) or Schwann cells (cells that wrap around nerves to improve the conduction of their signal) (Wang, et al 2016). Animal studies have shown that nerve conduits with added cells can be nearly as successful at promoting nerve regeneration in facial nerve injuries as nerve autografts (Wang, et al 2016) (Watanabe, et al 2017).

Animal studies on the use of these techniques to address facial nerve deficit have been promising (Masgutov, et al 2019). However, the potential for tumor growth when bone marrow or fat cells are isolated, cultured, and then reintroduced has limited the study and use of some of these treatments in the United States.

Nevertheless, cellular treatments may have the most exciting and substantial future for facial nerve regeneration. More research is needed before they can become more common in clinical use.

It's important to note that while many additional treatment options are being researched and approved for use by the United States Food and Drug Administration, the approval is based on safety—not effectiveness. These products include umbilical cord cells, amniotic membrane and fluid, and exosomes. Sometimes these treatments are falsely marketed as "stem cell" treatments, when actually they appear to be concentrated growth factors or signaling cells. (They nevertheless may be helpful to the body and the healing process.) These treatments are being used by different practitioners intraoperatively, by injection, and through intravenous infusion. However, there continues to be increased scrutiny surrounding their use, and new regulation and guidelines from the FDA are expected.

More and more, studies are confirming that regenerative medicine technologies are safe and effective for treating injuries and illnesses in various parts of the body—including the face. More research will increase our understanding of these techniques and ensure that the most effective approaches become available for patients who need them.

Hydrodissection and Other Ultrasound-Guided Procedures

Treatment for facial pain and palsy, as with most musculoskeletal conditions, may involve treating other areas of the body that are contributing to the problem.

Old injuries or weaknesses in your hip, sacroiliac joints, or shoulders can cause your body to react by increasing myofascial tension and the development of excess fibrous connective tissue called fibrosis. Over time, these areas of tension may restrict blood flow and nerve impulses and limit muscle movement and strength.

When myofascial tension builds at the base of the skull or occipital regions and around the temporomandibular (TMJ), or jaw joint, the nerves, blood flow, muscles, and tendon insertions of the face—which we use to close our mouth, smile, purse our lips, and raise, tighten, or close our eyelid—may be affected in some small or large way.

A nonoperative procedure called hydrodissection is proving to be effective at addressing these areas of tension and restriction.

Using ultrasound imaging, the restriction around an injured nerve can be located accurately and in real time. Fluid is then injected into the tissue to alleviate the tension, still under direct ultrasound guidance. This procedure is called ultrasound-guided percutaneous nerve hydrodissection.

Hydrodissection can also be used to affect tension due to scar tissue or adhesions in other musculoskeletal conditions. In ultrasound-guided percutaneous hydrodissection and debridement, which targets a muscle or tendon whose movement is limited by fibrosis, a needle is used to manually chisel and loosen up the restrictive tissue. In some cases, the offending matter then will be aspirated or removed.

Finally, in a procedure called a tenotomy, a needle can be used to manually fenestrate (poke tiny holes in) chronically diseased tendon tissue to stimulate healing.

More research is needed to determine the effectiveness and consistency of these approaches. But limited clinical results have been impressive: patients with paralytic facial conditions have reported significant improvements in strength, functionality, and pain relief.

CHAPTER 10

Acupuncture

Clayton Shiu, LAc, Phd

Can a medical intervention found to alleviate such ills as musculoskeletal pain, chronic headaches, and osteoarthritis also help mitigate Bell's palsy symptoms? Some studies of acupuncture—a Chinese modality practiced for thousands of years in the East, including to treat sudden facial palsy—suggest a qualified maybe, while legions of patients who've tried it say that acupuncture does, indeed, help.

If you haven't experienced acupuncture, you've no doubt seen pictures of it. During the procedure, a practitioner shallowly inserts short, thin needles into the client's skin at strategic points along pathways known as meridians. According to principles of Eastern medicine, "life energy" called qi (pronounced "chee") is said to circulate along some 20 meridians throughout the body. It is believed that this energy flows freely in healthy people; when it becomes blocked at any point, disease, illness, or pain can settle in. Inserting sterile needles, and sometimes adding heat or acupressure massage, at one or more corresponding points of impairment is believed to free the energy bottleneck and restore well-being.

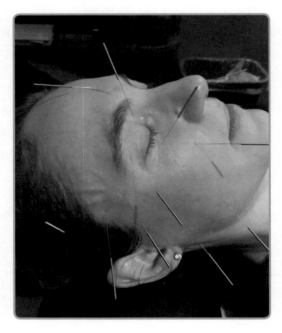

A patient receives acupuncture. The modality is endorsed by the World Health Organization for treating facial palsy during the first three to six months. Photograph courtesy of Clayton Shiu, PhD.

Beyond the idea of energy flow, acupuncture may work by affecting the body in several ways. One idea is that the micro-injuries created by the needles trigger the immune system to send healing, inflammation-reducing chemicals to the site. Another is that the simple act of being treated may induce the "placebo effect," a phenomenon whereby the patient believes the treatment can help, and so it does.

Here are some common questions about acupuncture as it relates to Bell's palsy.

What aspects of facial palsy can acupuncture help, and how?

Pain and inflammation. Multiple studies have found acupuncture to be an effective modality for reducing pain and inflammation, and some insurance plans cover the treatment.

Facial pain and stiffness are caused by inflammation, which results when circulation is bogged down by constricted blood vessels. Acupuncture can provide almost immediate relief by restoring proper blood flow through the affected area.

Acupuncture also has been shown to release serotonin, a pain-reducing endorphin in the brain. However, the relief is temporary.

Asymmetry. Physical and emotional stress are inextricably tied to Bell's palsy. Stress is considered in Eastern and Western medicine to be a risk factor for developing the condition. Acupuncture relaxes the patient and lowers their stress level, which can help ease muscle tension on the affected side and reduce the "off kilter" look that is the hallmark of facial palsy.

Fibrosis. The facial muscles of palsy patients who do not recover quickly can develop fibrotic tissue, a hard, sticky substance that forms when inflammation prevents fluid from circulating. The thick adhesions prevent the muscles from moving freely. A lopsided smile, for example, can result when fibrosis prevents the corners of the upper and lower lip from arching properly. So, even when damaged nerves have regenerated, they are unable to trigger the desired movement.

In Chinese medicine, fibrosis is considered a form of stasis, a stagnation of blood, fluid, phlegm, or even energy. Acupuncture practitioners may employ needles at trigger points along meridians thought to be related to neurological pathways. The resulting increase in blood flow, nerve firing, and immune system strength helps resolve the fibrosis.

How soon after onset can I try acupuncture?

Patients who receive the recommended medications upon onset (see Chapter 1) may be advised to wait one or two weeks to see if the condition stabilizes or begins to improve. Those who don't may wish to start treatment two or three days after onset.

Why do some people blame air conditioning or being outside in the freezing cold for causing their condition?

A time-honored theory holds that Bell's palsy is caused by exposure to cold and wind.

Here's the premise: When the face is exposed to lower temperatures and cold blowing air, the tissues stiffen. (Consider how water turns to ice when it's cold enough, and how the human body is mostly water.) This supposedly weakens the body, making a person more susceptible to facial pain or an attack of facial paralysis.

Testimonials linking cold to initial onset abound. One example is a patient who reported to his doctor that prior to getting Bell's palsy, he had been camping without the proper gear, sleeping on the cold ground on the left side of his face; a week later, he developed left-side facial palsy that took two months to heal. Posts blaming exposure to cold and wind—including air conditioning—are common on social media support groups for people with Bell's palsy.

Today, many acupuncturists view cold exposure as something that, in a predisposed person, can tip the scales toward what is thought to be the root cause of sudden facial palsy: reactivation of the virus behind cold sores (herpes simplex 1 virus) or chicken pox and shingles (varicella-zoster virus).

While this theory of exposure as a cause or contributing factor has not been proven by clinical studies, healthcare providers may nevertheless recommend that facial palsy patients avoid exposing their face to extreme cold and wind to prevent facial muscles from stiffening. They also cite the body's naturally lowered temperature during sleep as a reason why facial palsy symptoms may feel and appear worse upon waking.

What should I look for when choosing an acupuncturist?

At a minimum, your practitioner should have a master's degree in Chinese medicine from an accredited college or university. Ideally, they would have a background in neuroanatomy or postgraduate certification in rehabilitation techniques, particularly for stroke. Experience treating facial palsy patients is paramount.

The National Certification Commission for Acupuncture and Oriental Medicine provides a directory of NCCAOM practitioners at www.nccaom.org/find-a-practitioner-directory. Look for acupuncturist members with Dipl. Ac. licensure, awarded by state regulatory boards.

In general, beware of any acupuncturist who claims the ability to cure every medical condition.

Finally, a practitioner who follows an open-minded, integrated approach with Western medicine is best situated to achieve positive outcomes.

CHAPTER 11

The Emotional Impact of Unresolved Facial Palsy

Betsy Hirschel, LCSW-C

"There's my life before, and there's my life after. They are completely separate." —*Hannah*

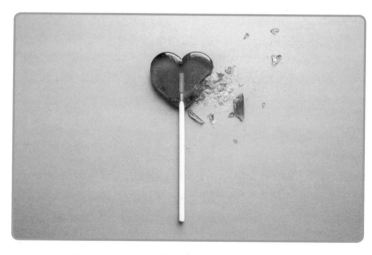

Photograph by Stas Knop / Shutterstock

Like the physical signs that commonly distinguish a person with facial palsy, emotional challenges are often part of the package.

Anger, sadness, embarrassment, and a host of other emotions can set in and wear away at even the most self-confident person. Physicians so regularly see depression and eroded quality of life among their patients with facial palsy that medical journal articles will often cite the condition's psychological impact along with its physiological elements.

Since your diagnosis, you've likely heard or read how "everyone's case is different." The same is true when it comes to processing and coping. One person may despair every time they look in the mirror or interact with someone; another may adopt an attitude like one woman who, after her recovery failed to progress, decided that her "cute little crooked smile" is simply "a cool anomaly I present to the world."

Still, there are experiences, feelings, and needs that many people with facial palsy share. We present them here with the caveat that this discussion may resonate most with those who are dissatisfied with their recovery.

Cancer Comparisons

Chances are you've heard, or felt, more than once how "you should be glad it's not cancer."

Of course you are. And gratitude for the health you do have is important. But this attempt at helping you deal with the trauma of facial palsy—whether someone says it to you, or you say it to yourself—belittles your own genuine struggle. It may even make you feel guilty for carrying negative emotions while other people are fighting life-threatening illnesses.

But others' challenges don't negate your own, and comparing bad situations is ultimately not constructive. Try to avoid getting mired in that trap.

Deniers

"Oh, you look fine. I couldn't even tell anything was wrong!"

If only you had a nickel for every time you've heard that, right?

People's well-intentioned attempts to make us feel better about our appearance can have the opposite effect when their words are disingenuous. After all, if half your mouth can't smile and one eye can't close, obviously something's wrong! So now we've got facial palsy *and* someone who's lying to us.

One woman who developed facial palsy from surgery for an acoustic neuroma remembers getting into a taxicab and noticing the driver staring at her. "What's wrong with your face?" he asked with curiosity, not unkindness. She was surprised to find that not only was she *not* offended, but she appreciated the driver's candor. They talked freely about her situation, even though she normally avoided discussing it.

Honesty—delivered compassionately—validates you. It makes you feel recognized, in more than just the physical sense. And *that* can be helpful.

Directors

Similar to the frustration of someone falsely claiming to not notice your facial palsy symptoms is the person who doesn't want *you* to notice or dwell on them, either. Because they can't identify with your situation—and usually because they want the best for you—they will try to direct you away from negative feelings by telling you to change your attitude. *"Just stop thinking about it." "Don't be so hard on yourself." "It's really not a big deal."*

This is not only counterproductive, but it's also a sign of disrespect to not acknowledge your right to feel. A more helpful response from them would be, "I'm sorry you are suffering," even if they honestly feel you have nothing to be despondent about.

Smile Police

When strangers see a person with facial palsy, they may read the downturn of an asymmetrical mouth as unfriendliness or sullenness. More than a few people have had their perfectly good mood ruined by a well-meant admonition to smile or cheer up. This happens to people who aren't affected by facial palsy, of course, but the unsolicited comment can land with extra force for someone who literally cannot just put on a happy face.

The Stranger in the Mirror

We tend to see ourselves in our mind's eye looking the way we prefer to look, the way we are accustomed to looking. This is not an issue of vanity; it's not a matter of feeling, or not feeling, handsome or pretty. But with lingering facial palsy, what you present to the world may look different than what you think you are presenting. "Who is that person, and where did I go?" is a common mental refrain. And with each glimpse in the mirror, each reflection in a storefront window, you are reminded of the disconnect between the you in your mind and the you others see. There is no getting away from it. This disconnect can be the biggest source of depression for some.

The Value of (Professional) Talk

"Maybe you should talk to someone" can be good advice when you're struggling to come to terms with negative emotions surrounding your condition. This struggle can manifest in many ways. For example, you might avoid social events or work opportunities; hide from your spouse, family, or close friends how facial palsy has affected your life; or worry that your partner is harboring their own negative feelings about your condition.

Psychologists (PhD) and licensed clinical social workers (LCSW), both of whom are frequently referred to as psychotherapists, can offer compassion and an empathic ear during psychotherapy. Pastors, rabbis, and other leaders at your house of worship may offer counseling as well.

Unlike physicians and physical therapists, who should have experience treating patients with facial palsy, a good psychotherapist doesn't need firsthand knowledge of it to be effective.

They need a nonjudgmental attitude, patience, and an ability to help people constructively navigate through their feelings. Sometimes, those feelings are buried or disguised as something else, such as self-deprecation, self-sabotaging behaviors, or anger directed at others. A good therapist can recognize this, respond with empathy, and help patients learn to trust and feel understood.

Therapy Concepts

Whatever your troubling feelings stemming from facial palsy may be, a good therapist won't tell you that you should or should not be feeling a certain way. (You may hear enough of that from well-meaning friends and family members.)

In fact, the first step a counselor may suggest is to take the word "should" out of your vocabulary.

> *"YOU WILL HEAL AND YOU WILL REBUILD YOURSELF AROUND THE LOSS YOU HAVE SUFFERED."*
>
> —ELISABETH KÜBLER-ROSS

"Should" is a shaming word, a finger-wagging word, when it comes to emotions. Feelings aren't right or wrong—they just are. Psychotherapists know this and won't tell you that you don't need to be angry at your situation. Instead, they will help you examine and process your feelings and experiences without denying or dismissing them.

Another therapy concept is learning to give yourself permission.

People with long-term facial palsy frequently experience grief and loss when their face is changed, and this grief can take on the appearance of sadness and depression. For many reasons, including family dynamics and societal or cultural norms, some people believe they are not entitled to feel this way. A psychotherapist can help you realize that not only are you allowed to feel your emotions, but that they are a normal, human reaction to experiencing such a significant loss. Our faces are what we present to the world and a big part of how we interact with others. If we are uncomfortable with what we are presenting, it can change those interpersonal dynamics. In addition, facial paralysis can affect some people's professions and passions: a broadcaster may not be able to appear on camera, for example, or a flutist may be unable to play their instrument. These would not be easy losses for anyone to face.

Add to these stressors the fact that people often believe grief and loss are things that need to be "gotten over" in a certain amount of time. But it's important to not only acknowledge the legitimacy of your loss, but to also give yourself permission to feel it for as long as it exists in you. You need not feel pressure, external *or* internal, to "get over it soon." It could be 16 months or 16 years, and that's okay. At the same time, a therapist can help you with strategies to avoid feeling stuck and learn how to move forward.

The late Elisabeth Kübler-Ross (1926–2004), a Swiss-American psychiatrist who pioneered concepts in death, dying, and stages of grief, wrote in her book *On Death and Dying*, "You will not 'get over' the loss … you will learn to live with it. You will heal and you will rebuild yourself around the loss you have suffered. You will be whole again but you will never be the same. Nor should you be the same nor would you want to."

Some people cannot tolerate the thought of talking one-on-one with a therapist. For them, group therapy can be an excellent way of connecting while staying in their comfort zone. Another potentially therapeutic step is to take part in one or more of the support groups for people with facial palsy on Facebook or other social media platforms. (Start by searching for keywords Bell's palsy, facial paralysis, Ramsay Hunt syndrome, or acoustic neuroma.) Many members say they find it cathartic to share with each other or even just read comments from people who know what they are going through better than anyone.

Coping Strategies

Facial palsy can intrude in many facets of life. Here are some suggestions that may help make things less troubling.

Ask for what you need! This might include steps such as asking your employer for flex time to accommodate physical therapy appointments, sending an overstuffed sandwich back in a restaurant because it's too difficult to eat, or asking a friend to help you blow out candles on a birthday cake.

Take a step back. We tend to be our own worst critics, and—unless your case was severe and your recovery was limited—it is possible that you perceive the anomalies in your face to be more obvious than others do. People who knew you before you got facial palsy may or may not be attuned to the changes, but it's far less likely that people you are meeting for the first time will immediately think "medical condition" when looking at you. With very few exceptions, we are all born with some degree of facial asymmetry.

Give a heads-up. If, however, facial palsy has made you self-conscious and convinced that people are judging your face, consider disclosing your condition up front. During a job interview, for instance, you might briefly explain what happened "in case you were wondering." If you do online dating, you might mention it in your profile, so you'll know that the people who reach out to you are already fine with your situation. But if you are not comfortable bringing up the topic, you don't have to. You don't owe anyone an explanation.

Find what works for you. Two particularly confident women decided to draw attention away from their facial palsy: one dyed her hair purple and silver, and the other wears tops that show off her cleavage! Another who felt her condition made her eyebrows look like they were "on two different continents," as she put it, got eyebrow tattooing for a more symmetrical appearance between the two. Other ideas:

- Grow facial hair to divert attention from a lopsided mouth.
- Change how you part your hair, or have your stylist cut long bangs. The stylist might also have good suggestions for changes that put the emphasis on features you like. Or, take the seemingly counterintuitive approach that one stylist came up with: she styled her client's long hair to cover her *unaffected* side! The client was thrilled to discover that the "bad" side didn't seem so afflicted when there was no "good" side to compare it to.
- Consult with a makeup artist or check out YouTube videos to learn effective techniques for improving symmetry with makeup.
- Try wearing glasses if you are bothered by an affected eye that appears smaller or squints from synkinesis. (If your vision doesn't need correction, you can get "plano" lenses, which don't have a prescription.) One person who tried this trick said the glasses emotionally felt like a "protective cover" that made her less tense when talking to people.

Seek the silly. If you can find something amusing or even absurd about your condition, the levity can make a real difference in how you feel—even if only temporarily.

One person who realized it had been a while since she found *anything* funny discovered that using curse words during her speech therapy exercises made her laugh and feel lighter. Another made the best of her eye patch by allowing her nephews to dress her as a pirate. And a third was able to laugh when the studio photographer who shot photos of her with her new grandson cropped off her head: she had to agree with the photographer that it was the most appropriate thing to do given that she inevitably would have been unhappy with how she looked. Best of all, the cropping resulted in an exquisite, artful picture.

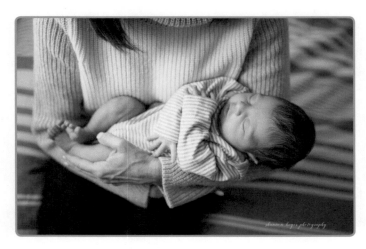

A cherished photo that is affectionately referred to by the family as "headless grandma." Photograph by Shannon Hager Photography.

To be sure, overall there is very little that is humorous about facial palsy. You may never find a single aspect of it that you can laugh at. You may, however, find something worthwhile emerging from the fog of your despondency.

Life repeatedly throws adversities our way, whether they are minor bumps in the road or full-blown traumas. Just like when we get a flat tire, we have to stop, figure out what's wrong, fix the problem, and move on. We can't stop these ruptures from occurring—a job will be lost, a marriage will be tested, an illness will emerge—but we can repair them to the best of our ability. Rupture, repair. Rupture, repair.

Doing this work, overcoming adversity, takes resilience. And it's from trauma that resilience is born.

INDEX

R

Radial pulse therapy 62
Ramsay Hunt syndrome i, ii, 3, 6, 7, 8, 9, 11, 21, 22, 36, 54, 55, 76, 79, 95, 101, 105
Reanimation, facial xiv, 46, 50, 52, 102
Recovery rates 4, 7, 37, 58
Regenerative medicine ix, 85, 87, 104
Rest 22, 25, 46, 49, 51, 56, 72, 103
Restylane® xvi, 44

S

Salivary glands 20
Self-esteem 13, 44
Selfies 18, 23
sEMG 58, 82, 83
Serotonin 90
Seventh cranial nerve ix, 3, 4, 5, 18, 19, 24, 25, 26, 36, 45, 85
Shingles 5, 6, 7, 8, 9, 18, 91
Sir Charles Bell 4
Smile vii, 2, 6, 11, 12, 13, 15, 24, 26, 36, 41, 43, 44, 46, 47, 48, 49, 50, 51, 52, 55, 58, 60, 64, 72, 74, 84, 87, 90, 92, 93, 94
Social media 91, 95
Sores 5, 8, 20, 21, 91
Speech 2, 12, 15, 20, 27, 44, 58, 64, 97
Static tissue repositioning 48
Steroids 7, 8, 11, 14, 18, 23, 38
Straws 19, 23
Stretching xiv, 67, 68, 69, 72, 73
Stroke xiv, 2, 3, 9, 14, 91
Support xi, xii, 12, 22, 64, 91, 95
Synkineedling® 60
Synkinesis 17, 21, 35, 36, 38, 39, 41, 46, 47, 55, 57, 58, 60, 61, 65, 66, 67, 68, 71, 72, 83, 96, 102

T

Tarsorrhaphy 34
Taste 2, 20, 25, 27
Tears xvi, 2, 15, 16, 25, 30, 31, 32, 33, 34
Telehealth 64, 65
Tendon transfer 50, 102
Tensor Fascia Lata 48
Temporomandibular joint disorder/TMD xi, xii, xv, 20
Transplant, muscle 48, 50, 51, 102
Trigeminal neuralgia 86, 103
Triggers, viral 5
Tumors v, 4, 6, 12, 87

U

Ultrasound xv, xvi, 21, 58, 59, 60, 61, 65, 83, 86, 87, 88, 103, 104

V

Vanity 94
Varicella-zoster virus 5, 91, 101
Vasopneumatic pump 62
Vertigo 2, 6
Vision 14, 16, 31, 34, 37, 44, 96
Vitamin B-12 21, 22

W

Wrinkles 27

X

Xeomin® 38, 66

Z

Zoster sine herpete 6, 55, 77
Zygomatic branch 25

BIBLIOGRAPHY

Chapter 1

Engström, M., T. Berg, A. Stjernquist-Desatnik, S. Axelsson, A. Pitkäranta, M. Hultcrantz, M. Kanerva, P. Hanner, L. Jonsson. 2008. "Prednisolone and Valaciclovir in Bell's Palsy: a Pandomised, Double-blind, Placebo-controlled, Multicentre Trial." *The Lancet Neurology* (11): 993-1000. DOI: 10.1016/S1474-4422(08)70221-7. Epub 2008. PubMed PMID: 18849193.

Lin, R.J., M. Klein-Fedyshin, C.A. Rosen. 2019. "Nimodipine Improves Vocal Fold and Facial Motion Recovery After Injury: A Systematic Review and Meta-analysis." *The Laryngoscope* 129 (4): 943-951. DOI: 10.1002/lary.27530. Epub 2018 Nov 19. PubMed PMID: 30450691.

Monsanto, R., A. Bittencourt, N. Neto, S. Beilke, F. Lorenzetti, R. Salomone. 2016. "Treatment and Prognosis of Facial Palsy on Ramsay Hunt Syndrome: Results Based on a Review of the Literature." *International Archives of Otorhinolaryngology* 20 (4): 394-400. DOI: 10.1055/s-0036-1584267 PubMed PMID: 27746846.

Sin, J.H., H. Shafeeq, Z.D. Levy. 2018. "Nimodipine for the Treatment of Otolaryngic Indications." *American Journal of Health-Systems Pharmacy* 15; 75 (18): 1369-1377. DOI: 10.2146/ajhp170677. Review. PubMed PMID: 30190294.

Sullivan, F.M., I.R. Swan, P.T. Donnan, J.M. Morrison, B.H. Smith, B. McKinstry, R.J. Davenport, L.D. Vale, J.E. Clarkson, V. Hammersley, S. Hayavi, A. McAteer, K. Stewart, F. Daly. 2007. "Early Treatment with Prednisolone or Acyclovir in Bell's Palsy." *The New England Journal of Medicine* 18; 357 (16): 1598-607. DOI: 10.1056/NEJMoa072006. PubMed PMID: 17942873.

Tang, Y.D., X.S. Zheng, T.T. Ying, Y. Yuan, S.T. Li. 2015. "Nimodipine-mediated Re-myelination After Facial Nerve Crush Injury in Rats." *Journal of Clinical Neuroscience* 22 (10): 1661-8. DOI: 10.1016/j.jocn.2015.03.048. Epub 2015 Jul 10. PubMed PMID: 26169537.

Weinberg, A., Z. Popmihajlov, K.E. Schmader, M.J. Johnson, Y. Caldas, A.T. Salazar, J. Canniff, B.J. McCarson, J. Martin, L. Pang, M.J. Levin. 2019. "Persistence of Varicella-Zoster Virus Cell-mediated Immunity After the Administration of a Second Dose of Live Herpes Zoster Vaccine." *The Journal of Infectious Diseases* 7; 219 (2): 335-338. DOI: 10.1093/infdis/jiy514. PubMed PMID: 30165651.

Azizzadeh, B. and J.L. Frisenda. 2018. "Surgical Management of Postparalysis Facial Palsy and Synkinesis." *Otolaryngologic Clinics of North America* 51 (6): 1169-78.

Azizzadeh, B., L.E. Irvine, J. Diels, W.H. Slattery, G.G. Massry, B. Larian, et al. 2019. "Modified Selective Neurectomy for the Treatment of Post-facial Paralysis Synkinesis." *Plastic and Reconstructive Surgery* 143 (5): 1483-96.

Bianchi, B., A. Ferri, V. Poddi, A. Varazzani, S. Ferrari, G. Pedrazzi G, et al. 2016. "Facial Animation with Gracilis Muscle Transplant Reinnervated via Cross-face Graft: Does It Change Patients' Quality of Life?" *Journal of Cranio-Maxillofacial Surgery* 44 (8): 934-9.

Bilyk, J.R., M.T. Yen, E.A. Bradley, E.J. Wladis, and L.A. Mawn. 2018. "Chemodenervation for the Treatment of Facial Dystonia: A Report by the American Academy of Ophthalmology." *Ophthalmology* 125 (9): 1459-1467. DOI: 10.1016/j.ophtha.2018.03.013. Epub 2018 Apr 10. Review. PubMed PMID: 29653859.

Byrne, P.J., M. Kim, K. Boahene, J. Millar, and K. Moe. 2007. "Temporalis Tendon Transfer as Part of a Comprehensive Approach to Facial Reanimation." *Archives of Facial Plastic Surgery* 9 (4): 234-41.

Engström, M., T. Berg, A. Stjernquist-Desatnik, S. Axelsson, A. Pitkäranta, M. Hultcrantz, M. Kanerva, and P. Hanner, L. Jonsson. 2008. "Prednisolone and Valaciclovir in Bell's Palsy: A Randomised, Double-blind, Placebo-controlled, Multicentre Trial." *The Lancet Neurology* 7 (11): 993-1000. DOI: 10.1016/S1474-4422(08)70221-7. Epub 2008 Oct 10. PubMed PMID: 18849193.

Marsk, E., N. Bylund, L. Jonsson, L. Hammarstedt, M. Engström, N. Hadziosmanovic, and T. Berg, M. Hultcrantz. 2012. "Prediction of Nonrecovery in Bell's Palsy Using Sunnybrook Grading." *The Laryngoscope* 122 (4): 901-6. DOI: 10.1002/lary.23210. Epub 2012 Feb 28. PubMed PMID: 22374870.

McAllister, K., D. Walker, P.T. Donnan, and I. Swan. 2013. "Surgical Interventions for the Early Management of Bell's Palsy." *The Cochrane Database of Systematic Reviews* (10): CD007468. DOI: 10.1002/14651858.CD007468.pub3. Review. PubMed PMID: 24132718.

Oyer, S.L., J. Nellis, L.E. Ishii, K.D. Boahene, P.J. Byrne. 2018. "Comparison of Objective Outcomes in Dynamic Lower Facial Reanimation with Temporalis Tendon and Gracilis Free Muscle Transfer." *JAMA Otolaryngology—Head & Neck Surgery* 144 (12): 1162-8.

Chapter 9

Banks, A.R. 1991. "A Rationale for Prolotherapy." *Journal of Orthopaedic Medicine* 13 (3).

Bennett, G.J., et al. 1988. "A Peripheral Mononeuropathy in Rat that Produces Disorders of Pain Sensation Like Those Seen in Man." *Pain* 33 (1): 87-107.

Cho, H.H., S. Jang, S.C. Lee, H.S. Jeong, J.S. Park, J.Y. Han, K.H. Lee, Y.B. Cho. 2010. "Effect of Neural-induced Mesenchymal Stem Cells and Platelet-rich Plasma on Facial Nerve Regeneration in an Acute Nerve Injury Model." *Laryngoscope* 120 (5): 907-13. DOI: 10.1002/lary.20860.

Doss, A.X. 2012. "Trigeminal Neuralgia Treatment: A Case Report on Short-term Follow Up After Ultrasound Guided Autologous Platelet-rich Plasma Injections." *Neurology* 3: 1-5.

Farrag, T.Y., M. Lehar, P. Verhaegen, K.A. Carson, P.J. Byrne. 2007. "Effect of Platelet Rich Plasma and Fibrin Sealant on Facial Nerve Regeneration in a Rat Model. *Laryngoscope* 117 (1): 157-65.

García de Cortázar, U., S. Padilla, E. Lobato, D. Delgado, and M. Sánchez. 2018. "Intraneural Platelet-rich Plasma Injections for the Treatment of Radial Nerve Section: A Case Report." *Journal of Clinical Medicine* 7 (2): pii:E13. DOI: 10.3390/jcm7020013.

Hashemi, Masoud, Parviz Jalili, Shirin Mennati, Alireza Koosha, Ramin Rohanifar, Firouz Madadi, Seyed Sajad Razavi, and Farinaz Taheri. 2015. "The Effects of Prolotherapy with Hypertonic Dextrose Versus Prolozone (Intraarticular Ozone) in Patients with Knee Osteoarthritis." *Anesthesiology and Pain Medicine* 5 (5).

Hibner, M., M.E. Castellanos, D. Drachman, and J. Balducci. 2012. "Repeat Operation for Treatment of Persistent Pudendal Nerve Entrapment After Pudendal Neurolysis." *Journal of Minimally Invasive Gynecology* 19 (3): 325-330. DOI: 10.1016/j.jmig.2011.12.022.

Hilton, J. 1879. "On rest and Pain." In *Jacobesen WHA* (ed): *On Rest and Pain,* 2nd edition. New York: William Wood & Company.

Kuffler, D.P. 2014. "An Assessment of Current Techniques for Inducing Axon Regeneration and Neurological Recovery Following Peripheral Nerve Trauma." *Progress in Neurobiology* 116: 1-12. DOI: 10.1016/j.pneurobio.2013.12.004.

Kuo, Y.C., C.C. Lee, and L.F. Hsieh. 2017. "Ultrasound-guided Perineural Injection with Platelet-rich Plasma Improved the Neurophysiological Parameters of Carpal Tunnel Syndrome: A Case Report." *Journal of Clinical Neuroscience* 44: 234-236. DOI: 10.1016/j.jocn.2017.06.053.

Levi-Montalcini, R., et al. 1982. "Developmental Neurobiology and the Natural History of Nerve Growth Factor." *Annual Review of Neuroscience* 5: 341-62.

Linetsky, F., K. Botwin, L. Gorfine, G.W. Jay, B. McComb, R. Miguel, et al. 2001. "Regenerative Injection Therapy (RIT): Effectiveness and Appropriate Usage." *Florida Academy of Pain Medicine (FAPM).*

Lyftogt, J. 2007. "Subcutaneous Prolotherapy Treatment of Refractory Knee, Shoulder, and Lateral Elbow Pain." *Australasian Musculoskeletal Medicine* 12 (2):110-12.

Masgutov, R., G. Masgutova, A. Mullakhmetova, M. Zhuravleva, A. Shulman, A. Rogozhin, V. Syromiatnikova, D. Andreeva, A. Zeinalova, K. Idrisova, C. Allegrucci, A. Kiyasov, and A. Rizvanov. 2019. "Adipose-Derived Mesenchymal Stem Cells Applied in Fibrin Glue Stimulate Peripheral Nerve Regeneration." *Frontiers in Medicine* 6:68. DOI: 10.3389/fmed.2019.00068.

Mohammed, Suja, and James Yu. 2018. "Platelet-rich Plasma Injections: An Emerging Therapy for Chronic Discogenic Low Back Pain." *Journal of Spine Surgery* 4 (1): 115-122.

Rabago, D., A. Slattengren, A. Zgierska. 2010. "Prolotherapy in Primary Care Practice." *Prim Care* 37 (1): 65-80.

Sánchez, M., T. Yoshioka, M. Ortega, D. Delgado, and E. Anitua. 2014. "Ultrasound-guided Platelet-rich Plasma Injections for the Treatment of Common Peroneal Nerve Palsy Associated with Multiple Ligament Injuries of the Knee." *Knee Surgery, Sports Traumatology, Arthroscopy* 22 (5): 1084-1089. DOI: 10.1007/s00167-013-2479-y.

Sánchez, Mikel, Ane Garate, Ane Miren Bilbao, Jaime Oraa, Fernando Yangüela, Pello Sánchez, Jorge Guadilla, Beatriz Aizpurua, Juan Azofra, Nicolás Fiz, and Diego Delgado. 2018. "Platelet-Rich Plasma for Injured Peripheral Nerves: Biological Repair Process and Clinical Application Guidelines, Demystifying Polyneuropathy." *Recent Advances and New Directions,* Patricia Bozzetto Ambrosi, IntechOpen, DOI: 10.5772/intechopen.81104.

Sayad Fathi, S., and A. Zaminy. 2017. "Stem Cell Therapy for Nerve Injury." *World Journal of Stem Cells* 9 (9): 144–151. DOI:10.4252/wjsc.v9.i9.144.

Seffer, I., and Z. Nemeth. 2017. "Recovery from Bell Palsy after Transplantation of Peripheral Blood Mononuclear Cells and Platelet-rich Plasma. *Plastic and Reconstructive Surgery Global Open* 5 (6): e1376. DOI:10.1097/GOX.0000000000001376.

Wang, T.V., S. Delaney, and J.P. Pepper.2016. "Current State of Stem Cell-mediated Therapies for Facial Nerve Injury." *Current Opinion in Otolaryngology & Head and Neck Surgery* 24 (4): 285–293.

Watanabe, Y., R. Sasaki, H. Matsumine, M. Yamato, and T. Okano. 2017. "Undifferentiated and Differentiated Adipose-derived Stem Cells Improve Nerve Regeneration in a Rat Model of Facial Nerve Defect." *Journal of Tissue Engineering and Regenerative Medicine* 11 (2): 362–374. DOI:10.1002/term.1919.

Weglein, Adam D. 2011. "Neural Prolotherapy." *Journal of Prolotherapy 3 (2): 639-643.*

Wu, Y.T., T.Y. Ho, Y.C. Chou, M.J. Ke, T.Y. Li, G.S. Huang, et al. 2017. "Six-month Efficacy of Platelet-rich Plasma for Carpal Tunnel Syndrome: A Prospective Randomized, Single-blind Controlled Trial." *Scientific Reports* 7(1): 94. DOI: 10.1038/s41598-017-00224-6.

Take Our Survey

The Foundation for Facial Recovery invites you to take a short, confidential survey about this book at:

www.foundationforfacialrecovery.org/survey.

Your feedback will help inform future education and research initiatives aimed at helping patients and healthcare providers overcome the challenges of facial palsy.

For more about the foundation, visit www.foundationforfacialrecovery.org.

Front cover: Photograph by Rohappy / Shutterstock

Back cover: At left, a 46-year-old patient presenting with Ramsay Hunt syndrome. Photograph courtesy of The Center for Facial Recovery. Right: Patient and her daughter 20 months later. Photograph courtesy of the patient.

Printed in the United States
By Bookmasters